**wellcome
collection**

WELLCOME COLLECTION publishes thought-provoking books exploring health and human experience, in partnership with leading independent publisher Profile Books.

WELLCOME COLLECTION is a free museum and library that aims to challenge how we think and feel about health by connecting science, medicine, life and art, through exhibitions, collections, live programming, and more. It is part of Wellcome, a global charitable foundation that supports science to solve urgent health challenges, with a focus on mental health, infectious diseases and climate.

wellcomecollection.org

THE
STORY
OF THE
BRAIN
IN 10½
CELLS

Richard Wingate

PROFILE BOOKS

wellcome collection

First published in Great Britain in 2023 by
PROFILE BOOKS LTD
29 Cloth Fair
London
ECIA 7JQ
www.profilebooks.co.uk

Published in association with Wellcome Collection

**wellcome
collection**

83 Euston Road
London NWI 2BE
www.wellcomecollection.org

10 9 8 7 6 5 4 3 2 1

Typeset by CC Book Production
Printed and bound in Great Britain by Clays Ltd, Elcograf S.p.A.

A CIP catalogue record for this book is available from the British Library.

ISBN: 978 1 78816 296 8
EISBN: 978 1 78283 576 9

For Flora, Thomas, Chloe and Bea

Contents

Acknowledgement

Science in practice is a conversation and I would like to acknowledge all the fantastic discussions with the brilliant – very brilliant – members of the small team that has been 'my' lab and with the friends who are so much more than simply colleagues.

If I have shaped any of the science to make a better story, maybe it is because, through stories, we make better science.

Preface

Any scientist sitting down to write a book that has any claim to a completeness – and a story does sound like it should be complete – has to issue an apology. It is in our nature to be cautious and even-handed, to weigh the evidence, highlight gaps and tentatively suggest a conclusion. But a story is different from a scientific report and for all the episodes that I include, I know that there will be a thousand important tales that could have been left behind.

A couple of years ago a friend, a writer and journalist from Portugal, gave me a book by a professor of European Literature, Winfried Sebald. I am not quite sure how she knew that I would be gripped by his writing, but the languid journey he described with a slight air of melancholy is a rich mix of history, revelation and storytelling that I would love to emulate. In *The Rings of Saturn*, Sebald wanders the by-roads of East Anglia, the countryside around the university where he worked, picking up the stories that flash through the landscape. A literary scholar would likely label it as psychogeography and maybe the story of the brain through its cells is exactly this – a stroll through recollections, my own and others.

The story of brain cells is tightly interwoven with the personalities of the people who described them. This isn't the way that science cultures evolve or how the history of science might be talked about these days, but brain cells have personalities and individual stories that change with each observer. And the observers' stories make the tale come to life. There are collisions: Fridtjof Nansen, the young Arctic adventurer with a passion for microscopy and a hungry intellect, meets Istvan Apáthy, the studious Hungarian who took twelve painstaking years to publish his studies. There are tales of scientists who die too young: Enrico Sereni, impatient to make new discoveries and reach his goals, with an acute sense of how little time he had; Otto Deiters, struggling for money and sick with typhus, who came so close to a brain cell theory years before others would claim its discovery; Walter Pitts, homeless at fifteen, the mathematician at the heart of the artificial intelligence revolution, who abandoned his work at the end of his twenties to read and drink heavily for his last ten years. And between these lives, two world wars that shook up the paths and expectations of young scientists and pushed them towards a new science, neuroscience: Francis Crick, Warren McCulloch, Edgar Adrian.

Stories matter. The neuroscience pioneers who found themselves on the wrong side of a narrative also found that their reputations suffered and their voices were silenced: Apáthy, Joseph von Gerlach and Camillo Golgi, who discovered the technical approach that heralded modern neuroscience. And the storytellers who were neither pioneers nor original thinkers, but who told a gripping tale, coined a phrase or drew a compelling picture: Lewellys Barker in Baltimore and Heinrich Waldeyer in Berlin had an enormous if unrecognised impact on the world. They gave us the word 'neuron' and that single, unmistakeable picture of a brain cell that we all recognise.

Places matter. So many stories converge around the damp basement laboratories of a Cambridge University emerging into the twentieth century and, more potently, the marine biology research labs, the Stazione Zoologica Anton Dohrn, in Naples. When I visit this place, at some point in the future, as I feel I have to, will I sense the ghosts of Richard Gregory, JZ Young, Sereni, Nansen, Apáthy? I can feel the sun on my face as I bob on the gentle waves of the Bay of Naples, casting my net for copepods. This dream of where I could get to, the stories woven by scientists before me and the stories that I will be able to tell, all keep me going back to the mysteriously beautiful brain cell.

People in this story

- Lord Edgar Adrian (1889–1977), British electrophysiologist (Nobel laureate)

- Istvan Apáthy (1863–1922), Hungarian zoologist and histologist

- Richard Avedon (1923–2004), American fashion and portrait photographer

- Lewellys F. Barker (1867–1943), American doctor and neuroanatomist

- Vladimir Betz (1834–1894), Ukrainian anatomist

- Valentino Braitenberg (1926–2011), German psychiatrist and cyberneticist

- Korbinian Brodmann (1868–1918), German neurologist

- Eduardo Caianiello (1921–1993), Italian theoretical physicist
- Pedro Ramón y Cajal (1854–1950), Spanish neurohistologist, medical doctor, pathologist. Brother of Santiago Ramón y Cajal
- Santiago Ramón y Cajal (1852–1934), Spanish neuroanatomist and founder of modern neuroscience (Nobel laureate)
- Francis Crick (1916–2004) British biophysicist and neuroscientist (Nobel laureate)
- Otto Deiters (1834–1863), German neuroanatomist
- René Descartes (1596–1650), French philosopher
- John Dolland (1706–1761), British lens maker who patented the achromatic lens that had been invented by a barrister, Chester Moore Hall
- August Forel (1848–1931), French psychiatrist, neuroanatomist and zoologist
- Rosalind Franklin (1920–1958), British biophysicist
- Sigmund Freud (1856–1939), Austrian neuroanatomist, founder of psychoanalysis
- Theodor Fritsch (1858–1927), Prussian neurophysiologist
- Camillo Golgi (1843–1926), Italian neuroanatomist and inventor of a staining technique (Nobel laureate)
- Richard Gregory (1923–2010), British psychologist
- Rainer 'Ray' Guillery (1929–2017), British neuroanatomist

- Charles Judson Herrick (1868–1960), founding editor of the *Journal of Comparative Neurology* and author of *The Brain of the Tiger Salamander*

- Wilhelm His (1832–1904), German embryologist

- Eduard Hitzig (1838–1907), Prussian neurophysiologist

- Alan Lloyd Hodgkin (1914–1998), British physiologist (Nobel laureate)

- Andrew Huxley (1917–2012), British physiologist and inventor (Nobel laureate)

- Tatsuji Inouye (1881–1976), Japanese ophthalmologist

- John Black 'JB' Johnston (1868–1939), American comparative neuroanatomist

- Immanuel Kant (1724–1804), German philosopher

- Cesare Lombroso (1835–1909), Italian physician and founder of criminology

- Keith Lucas (1879–1916), British electrophysiologist

- François Magendie (1783–1855), French physiologist

- Warren McCulloch (1898–1969), American philosopher, physiologist, neuroscientist and pioneer of cybernetics

- Egas Moniz (1874–1955), Portuguese neurosurgeon and pioneer of the lobotomy (Nobel laureate)

- Fridtjof Nansen (1861–1930), Norwegian neuroanatomist, polar explorer and champion of refugees (Nobel Peace Prize)

- Wilder Penfield (1891–1976), American-Canadian neurosurgeon

- Walter Pitts (1923–1969), American mathematician

- Jan Purkyně (1787–1869), Czech anatomist and physiologist
- Pío del Río-Hortega (1882–1945), Spanish neuroanatomist, pioneer of glial cell biology
- Arnold Bernard Scheibel (1923–2017), American neuroanatomist and physiologist
- Madge E. 'Mila' Scheibel (died 1976), psychotherapist and neuroanatomist
- Enrico Sereni (1900–1931), Italian neurophysiologist
- Charles Scott Sherrington (1857–1952), British physiologist (Nobel laureate)
- W. Stendell (dates unknown), zoologist who provided first description of the mormyrid fish 1914
- Rudolf Virchow (1821–1902), German anatomist, pathologist and politician
- Heinrich Wilhelm Gottfried von Waldeyer-Hartz (1836–1921), German anatomist
- Leonard Worcester Williams (1875–1912), American comparative anatomist and physician. Died in an accident in a lift at Harvard. His insightful work on the squid was forgotten, misquoted and discovered anew by JZ Young in the 1930s
- William Hyde Wollaston (1766–1828), British chemist and inventor
- John Zachary 'JZ' Young FRS (1907–1997), British zoologist
- Adolf Ziegler (1820–1899), Swiss clinician and anatomical model maker working with Wilhelm His.

My first cell

*If thought has shape,
what does it look like?*

My first brain cell was bright fluorescent yellow – made
so by a dye, Lucifer yellow, that I had injected into its
fleshy centre using a vanishingly small glass tube. I had been
randomly probing brain fragments, carefully dissected into
dishes and placed under a microscope, with a glass rod pulled
into a fine point in a miniature forge. Suddenly, after what
seemed like months of attempts, the sharp glass needle hit the
invisible centre of a brain cell, penetrated its thin membrane
– without for once tearing a gaping hole – and the dye, contained and bright, flowed outwards into the taut sphere that
is the cell's body and then into its elaborate, tree-like arms.

I watched it fill rapidly with colour. First the thick branches,
which then split, and divided again into twisting tendrils until
the smallest and most delicate twigs glowed. I flicked my
wrist on a metal dial to pull the glass needle away from the
cell and stared through the two eyepieces of the microscope
down to the square millimetre of brain, twenty centimetres
below and separated from my eyes by twenty or more stages
of optically engineered glass.

Near darkness. The room faintly illuminated by the
reflected intense blue light emanating from an ultraviolet bulb

caged in its metal housing. There was a humming from the electronics to my right, the faint smell of mechanical oil from the dials, shutters and switches on my microscope. The cell was symmetrical, beautiful, perfect.

What can we read from a natural form? If you look at a tree in all its variety of shapes and sizes, we can sense how its upward growth tells the tale of a struggle for light and space. We know what it is trying to achieve from the determination of its shoots to seek out a patch of sun. And later in its life, when fully grown, we also see the story of the battles it has fought. A tree on an exposed coastline, shaved flat on top and hugging the contours of a cliff, tells of past storms and the prevailing wind. You don't need to have witnessed these gales to know the direction that they invariably came from or guess at how strong they are – the branches have long since bent away from their force and tell their story.

What about the structure of a brain cell? Like the tree, you only have to ask the question: that's an interesting shape, why did it grow like that? The difference is that instead of sunlight, the brain cell is reaching for something different: perhaps this is information – its own version of sunlight – or maybe nourishment in the form of chemicals seeping through the gaps between cells. The quality of that shape, the nuance of its form, have meanings we can only guess at. And to a large extent, your guess is just as good as mine.

There are different kinds of brain cells, just as there are different species of trees in a forest. Even though each brain cell is unique, each species of brain cell has its own favoured connections, characteristic shape and its unique job. Above all, they are individual pieces of an architectural puzzle on a monumental scale whose stories woven together make up the story of the brain. The cells in this book are ten (and a half) landmarks in this story.

I want to encourage you to see the brain through its brain cells using only this small group of siblings out of a cast of thousands. In doing so, you walk the footsteps of early scientists who used the brain cell as the lens through which to see the workings of the mind. You also walk the path still trodden by contemporary scientists: by me and my friends, students and colleagues, as we peer into a microscopic world. The questions for me are still the same as with my first brain cell with its glowing, yellow, gently curving branches. What is it in the quality of information it carries that makes it grow this way? What is the meaning of this beautiful, elegant form?

There is a passage written by one of the early brain pioneers, Santiago Ramón y Cajal (1852–1934), that almost invariably moves me to tears. I use the quote in lectures to students quite often. It illustrates a landmark moment in the science of the brain and also a moment of personal revelation. It's the beautifully articulated instant in time when everything changes; for the brain, for Cajal himself. But as important as it is as a moment for science and for an unlikely scientific genius from a dusty and impoverished mountainside village, I still can't work out why it makes me cry and it has become a private joke with myself – a test. I make the point of reading it aloud whenever I can to a class. However hard I try, I hear the crack in my voice, a hoarseness in my throat and I have to turn away from the audience to read from the projector screen, hiding the emotion as best I can. I don't think anyone has noticed yet. And however often I test myself, the result is the same.

The passage marks a moment of revelation that is a turning

point for science – the start of one man's remarkable crusade to understand the brain through its brain cells but also a launch pad for a thousand more careers. Cajal was not the first person to look at the microscopic form of the brain, but his ability to empathise with what he saw and the imagination he brought to its understanding stood out among his peers.

The year that the passage was written was 1887. Santiago Ramón y Cajal was the director of the Anatomical Museum in Zaragoza, a veteran soldier of the Cuban campaign and a doctor who had just lived through a terrifying cholera epidemic with his young family in Valencia. His career had been tortuous: a failed high school education, an apprenticeship to a barber, then to a shoemaker, back to high school and finally a half-hearted journey through medical school, spending his time writing fiction and verse, reading philosophy and building up his physique through weights and obsessive exercise. After military service and a near-fatal illness, he had claimed his doctor's licence and finally established himself with a wife and children, gained a position in a medical school, and discovered a passion for microscopes.

When cholera followed Cajal from Valencia to the city of Zaragoza, he threw himself into the unfolding public health crisis, devising a new and rapid way of detecting its pathogen in human samples. In gratitude, the city gave a gift of a modern, gleaming microscope that allowed him to indulge his obsession. With his new instrument, Cajal set up a small laboratory at home where he could both conduct research and perfect his skills with microscopy by systematically studying the tissues in the body.

He had left the investigation of the brain until last, knowing that its impenetrable complex tangle made any sensible decoding of its structure almost impossible. However, as he started to explore neural tissue, even the smallest insight into this uncharted realm delighted him. Isolated from the resources and libraries in the mainstream science powerhouses of Germany and France, he had to scrape together money for subscriptions to journals and tried every technique that they described using the tools and chemical reagents at hand.

A pivotal turning point in his life came with a chance trip to the capital of Spain. With his status in the academic world secured, Cajal was invited to sit on an interview panel for candidate anatomy teachers in Madrid. He took the opportunity to visit colleagues in what can best be described as an informal biology 'salon' – a hobbyist's laboratory that, like Cajal's own laboratory in Zaragoza, had been squeezed into a house in Calle de la Gorguera,[i] a few steps from the Plaza de Santa Ana. This was an era in Spain when the idea of conducting research that could be written about or published in journals was a seemingly impossible dream to Cajal. Exploration of this kind was certainly not part of the Spanish anatomist's day job. In the salon, ideas could be discussed and experiments conducted away from the formal corridors of the medical school. The excitement was infectious.

It was in this clubhouse atmosphere that Cajal met Luis Simarro, a neurologist who had only recently returned from Paris and who was fired up with enthusiasm for the new research he had seen. Better still, he had brought back some of the material that he had encountered in his travels. Simarro invited Cajal back to his own home, and his private microscope, to show him some of the treasures that he had gathered. Among the samples, brightly coloured, glued with gum to slides, cut into thin or thick slices, one blackened lump of brain stood out. It was prepared using a technique invented in Pavia by Camillo Golgi. Simarro even had a rare copy of some of the drawings its inventor had made and recipes for the technique published in a memoir just one year before.

What Cajal saw next in Simarro's back-room laboratory changed his life. He could not sleep that night and early the next morning he was knocking again on Simarro's front door to beg another look at a lump of brain chemically treated with what became known as the Golgi stain.

Against a clear background stood black threadlets, some slender and smooth, some thick and thorny, in a pattern punctuated by small dense spots, stellate or fusiform. All was sharp as a sketch with Chinese ink on transparent Japan-paper. And to think that that was the same tissue which when stained with carmine or logwood left the eye in a tangled thicket where sight may stare and grope ever fruitlessly, baffled in its effort to unravel confusion and lost for ever in a twilit doubt. Here on the contrary, all was clear and plain as a diagram. A look was enough. Dumbfounded, I could not take my eye from the microscope.[1]

The words sound fresh to my ears and the experience of being dumbfounded, the jaw dropping, the blink to look again . . . that is the moment when you realise that here is something new, never seen before or seen by only a few.

My jaw dropped when I saw my first brain cell, emerging from the dark. It looked like rivers of molten metal being poured into a mould. That time I was frozen in awe, while other times I've jumped up and punched the air or paced the room trying to contain myself before looking again to make sure. These moments make up the best parts of science. Years of failed experiments can be forgotten in a moment. So Cajal's words reach into that part of me that makes me want to go back again and again to the raw excitement of discovery.

But there was more to this than just an excitement at a new tool or a glimpse of what next month's project might be at home in his own back-room lab. What Cajal witnessed in the house on Calle del Arco de Santa Maria[ii] was an answer, or rather the roadmap to an answer of the riddle of the brain itself. This was the dramatic and sudden unveiling of its architecture – a diagram that was yet without meaning, but for the first time, a richly filled canvas with structure and signposts. Cajal knew that the brain and its secrets were there for the taking. He returned home to Zaragoza and set off on a journey of discovery that changed his life and established the foundation of a science of the brain.

Brain cells are beautiful. They are compelling and varied in the same way that trees have a sinuous and emotional beauty. Trees have a form that speaks of their fight against gravity and wind to stretch into the light and grow. Brain cells have an identical, purposeful form but their nature and their variety have a purpose that we don't fully understand. The brain cell is the stuff from which the brain's function is built. Its shape is nothing less than the physical manifestation of a fragment of thought.

This was the realisation that stopped Cajal in his tracks. There, sitting at Luis Simarro's microscope, what sprang out of the blackened, dehydrated brain, drenched in silver and osmium, was a glimpse of the hidden language of all that we think and feel. He had imagined this moment before, in Zaragoza, as he had experimented and dissected, teased with forceps, dipped and stained tissue through one solution after another. But he never dreamed it would be like this: so clear, so sharply etched. Here was a pattern, a structure, wonderful and mysterious and pregnant with meaning waiting to be uncovered. All he needed to do was to look.

Cell 1

*Purkinje's cell and
the method of silhouettes*

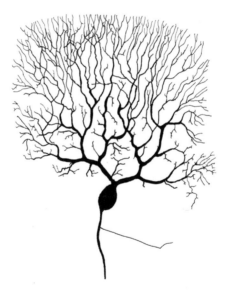

The completely flat Purkinje cell seen face on. Turned ninety degrees, it almost disappears from view. Its arcing and branching dendrites extend from a cell body up towards the surface of the brain. Its axon stretches down, extending out of the drawing, with, in this case, a single short branch close to the cell body. When Jan Purkyně first saw these brain cells, only the large round cell body and the thick trunk at the base of the dendritic tree were visible using the techniques available to him at the time.

The long journey from student to scientist is a peculiar rite of passage. It is a research apprenticeship that involves the production of a doctoral thesis – a body of work based on personal research. It sounds imposing and academic, and although libraries and journals are a part of the process, the hidden side of the thesis is the accumulation of strategies for coping with boredom and repetitive tasks, finding excitement and reward in the most obscure achievements. It is also a personal odyssey. Most people who undertake it experience an intensity of loneliness, frustration and indignation that far outweighs the unexpected moments of pleasure and excitement. My loneliest moments were spent in the dark with brain cells.

I spent four years sitting in front of a pool of projected light. Tracing the form of brain cells that I had photographed using a camera and a microscope. Piecing together their form. Joining dots to make coherent branches until the whole emerged. I did this for hundreds of brain cells, experiencing an unsettling disembodiment – just me, the pool of light and a radio, tuned at the time to news reports of the first Gulf War.

The laws of optics dictated that I would spend a large chunk of my life assembling pictures of whole cells by looking at a series of photographic negatives of the same picture, each with only a little piece of the scene in sharp focus. This is one of the unavoidable consequences of looking into the microscopic world. As the precision of lenses and their ability to resolve the finest details increases, their ability to capture anything above or below a very narrow vertical depth – anything 'out of focus' – disappears into a blur. Reconstructing the scene under the microscope with depth requires images being captured in multiple optical slices to build up a composite of the hidden world in sharp relief. If a brain cell stretches up and down through three dimensions, then tens or hundreds of images are needed to capture all its details.

These laws of optics have proved to be extremely useful. Sharply focused optical slices allow the three dimensions of the microscopic world to be reconstructed. This approach was first exploited in the late 1880s when a Swiss physician, Adolf Ziegler (1820–1899), teamed up with an embryologist, Wilhelm His (1832–1904). Together they transferred drawings of the outlines of series of slices through developing frogs, chickens and humans onto thin wax sheets. The wax sheets were then trimmed to match the traced outlines and layered on top of each other in the same alignment as the tiny slices from which they had been copied. Assembled in the correct order and with their rough edges smoothed into a seamless surface, the fully three-dimensional embryo emerged hundreds of times enlarged. These were giant embryos that could be held in two hands and passed between investigators and Ziegler's models proliferated throughout anatomy teaching labs the world over. They can still be found on dusty shelves in anatomy classrooms – rarely used today and a largely unrecognised and uncelebrated landmark of scientific discovery.

The wax slabs of His and Ziegler anticipated the techniques used today by a hundred years. In place of slices of wax, optical slices are taken and fed into digital three-dimensional reconstructions of anything from microscope images to magnetic resonance imaging scans. The three-dimensional voxels making up the 'volume' or 'stack' are the currency of biomedical imaging. Vast tera-bytes of storage are given over to reconstructing fractions of a millimetre of brain.

Back in the darkness, my cell drawings were still a few years away from being replaced by these digital innovations. I could use only old-fashioned celluloid film to capture the fragmented views of cells. The brain cells I was interested in were mercifully flat but even then, I dreaded depth. Any deviation from flatness meant a multiplication in the number of images I would be scanning by eye to make each drawing. Each of my photographic negatives captured thin slices with a fragment of a brain cell – the rest was a blur. I would slide a negative into position and its projected image would fall onto a piece of A4 paper. Scanning the image, sharp black edges indicated the brightest and sharpest form. I would trace these in pen and ignore the rest: perhaps only a single short line, a branch or a minute twig given by a single negative before moving to the next negative and the next focal plane.

The whole process of photography, developing negatives, mounting film strips in the enlarger and meticulous drawing seemed to me to have a reassuring sense of objectivity. By contrast, early microscopists drew what they saw as they looked down the single eyepiece of their microscope, sketching with one hand while adjusting the focus with the other. Working their way up and down the vertical planes they would mentally piece together in a freehand drawing what I was doing by my careful tracing. I was being more mechanical, more objective. My bet to myself was that if I was to repeat the process I had come up with, using the same set of negative images of the same cell, I could draw an identical picture again and again.

But that is not the way it worked out. Several times I found that I had unintentionally reconstructed the same brain cell twice. The same multiple negatives, the same pool of light, but two drawings that were subtly different. In the shifting of the paper, the flick of the pen, the guesses that bridged two sharp dots separated by a blur, in the incremental flow of the thickening branches and the finest of spines, something subjective crept into my method. Imagination was an essential ingredient to the way I was working. Which was the 'right' drawing? With practice, my drawings became more compelling, and more true to life. I realised they exhibited not just a modicum of artistic licence but also an artistic style.

What is artistic style when you are essentially tracing an outline? Something seeps into the way your hand moves after you have drawn brain cells again and again. Something about the energy of the way in which they have grown transfers into the drawings to give them life. I can tell immediately if a drawing is second-hand, penned by a professional illustrator copying from another source. There is something lifeless in the execution and the intention of the lines. The intuitive sympathy with the form is gone. To draw is to know. And for this reason, drawing became central to the development of brain cell theory. There is art at the heart of this science.

The first drawings of a bona fide brain cell were made in 1832. The cells that were depicted were a partial picture – a shadowy hint of what the brain contained – but important enough to bear their discoverer's name to this day.

Born in 1787, Jan Purkyně (Purkinje) was a Czech biologist working at the sharp edge of technology with a revolutionary new microscope. It incorporated an optical breakthrough, seized on by Peter Dolland, the son of John Dolland, a Huguenot refugee and former silk weaver in Spitalfields in London, who set up a glass factory in 1750. Together, father and son patented ingenious fusions of glass that could remove the rainbows that frustratingly blurred the edges of stars and planets viewed through telescopes and at the outlines of forms under the microscope. The sandwiches of glass compensated for the different angles of diffraction of different colours of light extinguishing the rainbowed fringes produced by more conventional instruments. The Dollands made increasingly sophisticated 'corrected' achromatic and apochromatic lenses that could now be incorporated into microscopes. In Breslau, Jan Purkyně, Professor of Physiology and Pathology, was one of the few scientists with enough financial backing to instal this revolutionary innovation in his laboratory in 1832. Armed with this new tool, he immediately set about describing what he saw in thin, hand-cut slices of preserved brain.

What was to become Purkyně's cell was glimpsed in its partial state, almost as a shadow, in a chunk of material from the cerebellum; the 'little brain' that sits below and to the back of the cerebral cortex. The surface of the cerebellum is like thick ribbon that has been folded repeatedly to make a compressed sandwich of undulating peaks and troughs, called 'folia'. If you were to cut across the ribbon, you would see that the folia are divided into clear layers. To Purkyně's eyes, the outermost layer was greyish, the inner layer was yellow, and where they met a string of fig-like 'corpuscles' seemed to extend short, stubby arms up towards the surface of the brain. His drawings of these corpuscles, which would later become known as the Purkinje cells, are now acknowledged as the first representation of brain cells.

Jan Purkyně's interpretation of what he had drawn was heavily influenced by the knowledge of cells in other organic forms of the natural world. The concept of cells – or more broadly the idea that plants and animals were built of cells of different shapes and sizes – was well established for all biological structures. Purkyně was confident in his description of this new entity within the brain that it was clearly a cell body with a distinct nucleus. However, there was only a single line of these 'corpuscles' that traced the boundary between yellow and grey layers undulating under the surface of the cerebellum. Where were the other cells of the brain? His theory was that the Purkinje cells were a collecting point for a mesh of convergent energy within the cerebellum, harvesting forces from a swirling sea of fibres all around.

But Purkinje cells were, in fact, not alone in the cerebellum and the full beauty of what lay at the end of the stubby arms, stretching upwards to the surface of the undulating ribbon of cerebellum, eluded him. Fifty years later, when Camillo Golgi of Pavia and then Santiago Ramón y Cajal of Madrid were able to ink the complete outline of the cell, the stubby arms that Purkyně had drawn proved to be only the trunks of what emerged as elaborate, intricately branching trees. The layer of corpuscles described by Purkyně were the anchor for wafer-thin filigrees of miniature branching fronds that were completely flat, arranged in parallel wafers and stacked upon each other in a delicate lattice sandwich.

However, as Golgi and Cajal completed their respective versions of the Purkinje cell, the seeds were sown for an extraordinary and notorious episode in the story of the brain. The drawings themselves became central to one of the most public and polarised scientific disagreements in the history of neuroscience.

On one side of the disagreement sat Camillo Golgi: the inventor of the eponymous revolutionary stain, which he called the 'black reaction' and which others nicknamed the method of silhouettes. It is a chemical process, with far-reaching significance for neuroscience, which unlocked the workings of brain cells in the late 1800s. On the other side was Cajal – an instinctive and dedicated convert to the method of silhouettes who understood how Golgi's technique had revealed something astonishing, which Golgi himself denied: that brains are built from cells.

The discovery of the black reaction by Golgi was a product of trial and error – an experimentation by candlelight with chemicals borrowed from the photographic darkroom. It would indelibly stamp Golgi's name on the most revolutionary technique ever seen in neuroscience but ironically leave his intellectual legacy in tatters.[2]

Golgi was born in Brescia in 1843 and followed in his father's footsteps to study medicine at the University of Pavia, where he became a pathologist. Here he worked as assistant to Cesare Lombroso (1835–1909), the controversial physician who believed that a whole range of human traits (including, notoriously, criminal behaviour) could not only be inherited but also be tracked by physical characteristics. Lombroso convinced Golgi that the material basis of mental disorders could be understood at the level of the microscope.

Despite promising first steps in the pathology laboratory, financial pressures forced Golgi to abandon Pavia and take a position as a physician and surgeon in Abbiategrasso on the outskirts of Milan. This relegated his research to an improvised laboratory, experimenting with just a few instruments, isolated from scientist colleagues and working through the night in a converted kitchen.

However, within a year, his first brief reports showed stunning new images. Golgi had taken potassium bichromate and mixed it with silver nitrate, emulating the recipe of the newly invented photographic developer solution, and applied it to the brain. Perhaps Golgi had hoped to develop a picture of mental processes, perhaps even an image of the outside world frozen on the brain's surface. Instead, what gradually condensed in preserved brain pieces were the black twigs and spindrels of cells. In the right conditions, an entire cell from the brain would emerge as an intact, coherent whole; branching, twisting, intricate and beautiful. Within three years his discoveries landed him a permanent job in Pavia and four years later, in 1879, he became Professor of Histology (the study of microscopic structure), publishing his own atlas of the microscopic structure of the brain, packed with beautiful hand-drawn plates, in 1885.

The truly miraculous fluke that made Golgi's black reaction into a transformative discovery was its random nature. In a sea of grey, a treated piece of brain might be filled with crisscrossing spindrels, or standing alone, a single perfect brain cell seemingly completely and definitively stained while others remain invisible. Suddenly the tangled mess – the landscape that Cajal had described as a territory for futile exploration – disappeared.

Of all the cells of the brain that can suddenly emerge from a Golgi stain, the Purkinje cell is undoubtedly one of the most startling. It is distinctive, instantly recognisable, arranged with its neighbours in an orderly row and organised in a way that can only speak to a precise function in information processing. Most of all, its 'cell-ness' cannot seemingly be denied. And by chance, the Purkinje cell is seen at its best in a slice that cuts at right angles across the crushed ribbon of folia that make up the cerebellum. Where Purkyně had seen a line of fig-shaped corpuscles with stubby arms stretching upwards, both Camillo Golgi and Santiago Ramón y Cajal saw an elaborate and highly branching tree with multiple fronds – a undeniably sensuous form. The tree that branched upwards and outwards, cut off at the trunk in Purkyně's view, but now magnificently revealed, came to be called the 'dendritic tree', each individual branch a 'dendrite'.

Golgi and Cajal, armed with the same tools, set off to draw the same cells. And at this moment Cajal made a transform-ative imaginative leap. As he looked at the dendritic tree he realised that the form of the brain cell dictated nothing less than a one-way channel for the flow of information. Much the same as Purkyně, he saw that the dendrites of Purkinje cells must be collecting something. With the power of the black reaction suddenly revealing dendrites throughout the brain in different cells, he reasoned that what they were collecting was information itself. If information was traced out in the converging branches of dendrites it followed that it was flowing like a stream to the origin of the tree – the cell body. What next? Emerging from the opposite side of the cell body to the dendritic tree, in nearly every brain cell he looked at, and in none more clearly than in the Purkinje cell, a single, stouter and smoother cellular root emerged. This was the output, later to be named the axon, through which the collected information from dendrites could be sent onwards to other cells.

This transfer of information from dendrites to cell body to axon became Cajal's law of dynamic polarisation – a theory of information flow in the brain that proved robust, complete and accurate. It transformed a static microscopic architecture of brain cells into a dynamic picture of rivers and tributaries of thought in the brain. It was a compelling vision. But Golgi, on whose invention Cajal had relied, disagreed.

The disagreement flared into the most public of scientific arguments in Stockholm in December 1906, when the Nobel Prize in Physiology or Medicine was given to both Santiago Ramón y Cajal and Camillo Golgi in the Nobel Foundation's first-ever joint award. The rules of the Nobel Foundation demanded that both men attend Stockholm in person and this gave the opportunity for special seminars in the days after the awards ceremony presided over by the King of Sweden. Cajal spoke first and delivered a beautifully illustrated lecture describing almost twenty years of painstaking reconstruction of the nervous system through its brain cells. He paid fulsome tribute to the discovery of the black reaction by Golgi, whom he had met for the first time just a few days earlier.

On the following evening, sitting in the audience to listen to Camillo Golgi, Cajal had expected the same recognition and the same effusive acknowledgement of the other scientific pioneers of what became known as a neuron doctrine, some of whom were sitting in the audience with Cajal.[i] What he heard shocked him to his core and left him trembling with impatience as he realised he had no way to correct a catalogue of errors and mistruths that flowed from a show of intolerable self-importance. Golgi systematically ignored the work of his rival scientists and focused instead on purely his own discoveries.

As he spoke, Golgi slowly and painstakingly dismantled the reputation that he had built for himself. It was a speech that in the space of a scientific seminar chipped away at his life's work and its legacy. What had initially seemed poor scientific etiquette in a failure to give credit where credit was due, became a shocking realisation for his audience that Golgi did not believe that brain cells existed. The idea that Golgi steadfastly promoted that evening was that the brain was a vast interconnected web of seamlessly joined fibres. The existence of individual cells was an illusion.

Where Cajal saw the microscopic architecture of information flowing along dendrites, Golgi saw root-like 'protoplasmic extensions' that sucked nutrients from the dense network of minute blood vessels that filled the brain. For him, the elaborate dendritic tree played no part in organising thought. Instead, its role was to support the function of the axon, which Golgi named the 'nerve fibre'. And here again Golgi diverged from Cajal. Where Cajal saw discrete wires that could each be traced back to an individual cell, Golgi described a fused mesh of fibres, similar to the hyphal tubes of a fungus. Like a fungus, the cellular structure of the brain was one continuous organic network. No element within this network could ever act individually and Cajal's universal law of dynamic polarisation was a sham. As Golgi continued in his speech, stunning his audience into mute astonishment and completely contradicting Cajal's theories laid out the previous evening, he saw no reason 'even now to abandon the idea which I have always insisted on'.[3]

How did two excellent observers and draughtsmen, working with the same material and the most advanced optical microscopes of their day, come up with such radically different conclusions about the form of the brain? As the audience listened, it became increasingly clear that the reasons for the disagreement lay in the finest details of the equally beautiful drawings that both Cajal and Golgi had made. At first glance, these drawings seemed identical.

All those years later, as I sat in front of the pool of light, drawing cells, I wondered about the errors that pen and ink might introduce and the reliability and reproducibility of evidence. I knew that if I tried to draw the same cell twice from my sequence of negatives, I would always end up with a subtly different image. But I would never draw cells as interconnected and even if the gap between them was small, its existence was never doubted. In other words, it would be impossible to imagine any other solution. And that was due to Cajal and his doctrine, telling me that there was such a thing as a brain cell.

However, for Golgi and Cajal there were no pre-existing doctrines and theories, only hints from other parts of nature: cells in other tissues, the hyphae of mushrooms and the vaguely sketched form made by Jan Purkyně fifty years before. Where Golgi saw dendrites collecting nutrients, Cajal saw dendrites gathering information. When Golgi saw nerve fibres close to each other, his pen joined the dots. Cajal, with the exact same material, did not. He left a critical, defining gap. That pause, where the pen momentarily lifted from the paper rather than completing a line, separated not only brain cells but marked the divergence of the reputation and legacies of the two scientists on that December evening in Stockholm. Cajal became an extraordinary, enduring influence on the field of neuroscience while Golgi retreated scientifically, leaving his name to the structures he discovered but no lasting intellectual fame. To me, sitting and drawing my own cells in the dark, these minute but fateful discrepancies in the pen touching the paper were not conscious decisions but a projection of what I imagined was there. When they drew, I know that Golgi and Cajal were imagining different things.

What shapes imagination? It is tempting to try to trace back the life stories of Golgi and Cajal, both sons of doctors and with superficially similar upbringings. Golgi grew up in an Alpine village near the Swiss border surrounded by steep pine-forested slopes. Cajal was born into the wooded hills of Navarra, for centuries an independent kingdom, but now a newly incorporated state in Spain. I like to think of Golgi as having a well-mannered upbringing in a family that was both financially comfortable and respectable. By contrast, Cajal forged a rebellious and adventurous childhood and, I feel, knew trees from intense personal experience. He ran wild through ancient oak woods shooting arrows at sparrows and hunting for birds' nests. He would play truant for hours, once for several days and, most importantly, climbed trees. I can see him clambering branch by branch, testing the weight tentatively with a foot or a hand, embracing the trunk, until craning to look and reaching a hand up to lift the magpie's nest, trying to catch a glimpse of the young hatchlings.

If all this disturbs that sense of the scientific and sounds too personal, too absurd, Cajal would be the first to agree that the subjective, the personality, explicitly shapes observation. My own anxiety at the small imaginative steps and traces of artistic style that crept into my drawings were not some kind of failing or cheating. On the contrary, the subjective sympathy with the object – an artistic resonance with what made sense – was a necessary way of expressing knowledge and understanding. Feeling the way along a tree as you climb is an understanding of how its form makes sense. This was the difference, in my imagination, that separated Cajal and Golgi making one reputation and condemning the other. As Cajal wrote much later, however hard you may try to be objective all there is ultimately is you, the author.

So what do Purkinje cells do and what is the function of the folded sheet that houses them – the cerebellum? In many ways, it is one of the simplest brain regions to explore, divided into layers with Purkinje cells sandwiched in the middle, and yet, ironically, is still one of the most mysterious.

Damage the cerebellum and a constellation of problems arise – most notably the unsteadiness on your feet, a tremor that gets worse as you try to pick something up and maybe even a drunken-sounding slur in your speech. The cerebellum is both a learning machine and an instantaneous error detector and when it is broken its importance in helping you move becomes painfully clear. Modern imaging techniques show that the cerebellum loves novelty or surprise and many years of studies have shown that it learns from mistakes. Disable your cerebellum and you will never be able to learn to play the piano.

Hidden by these outward signs are the more subtle shifts in cognitive and possibly emotional function. And it is these disorders of thought that predominate when the cerebellum is damaged in the unborn. Here, setbacks during pregnancy might result in problems in learning and communication, whereas movement is largely unaffected. In the rare cases where someone is born without a cerebellum, the function of the brain is apparently normal. The brain can learn to live without a cerebellum but cannot do without it when it is there.

Purkinje cells and their remarkably precise alignment in a regular geometry lie at the heart of this machine and maybe hold a clue to the function of the cerebellum. The stunningly regular arrangement and precision of Purkinje cell dendritic trees were the obsession of an Austrian scientist who argued that the cerebellum is the brain's stopwatch. Valentino Braitenberg (1926–2011) was only nine years old when Cajal died in 1934 at the age of eighty-two. He grew up speaking both Italian and German, completed a medical degree in Rome, but then decided to study the brain. In 1954, Braitenberg met Eduardo Caianiello (1921–1993), a theoretical physicist from Naples, at a seminar by the American mathematician Norbert Wiener, a pioneer of robotic control and computer systems. Both men were fascinated by Wiener's ideas and Caianiello persuaded the young doctor to help him to establish an institute of cybernetics in Naples.

Braitenberg's self-described approach to neural architecture was to think about the texture of the brain.[ii] Take a step back to view the whole population and Purkinje cells have a distinct texture of their own. Remember that they are flat and are lined up in parallel to the curves of the folded ribbon of the cerebellum, sandwiched between layers. Seen from the side, in a slice that cuts across the ribbon, this would look like a forest of trees rising with hills, falling into valleys, bending with the peaks and troughs of the folds. Now, rotate this scene by ninety degrees in your imagination and what happens? The lavish trees of dendrites disappear and, in their place, are pencil-thin lines, erect profiles of the flat Purkinje cell trees. Running through them, at right angles to this picket line of Purkinje cell flattened trees, are thousands upon thousands of axons bringing in information about body position, vision, hearing and movement.

Braitenberg was fascinated by the geometry of this arrangement. He calculated that if you could unfold the folded sheet of cerebellum the ribbon would be ten centimetres wide but more than a metre long. Running across this metre of ribbon are thousands of repeating lines of Purkinje cells feeding millions of inputs. The tiny gap between each neighbouring, flattened dendritic tree is remarkably similar from cell to cell. This, Braitenberg reasoned, gives the cerebellum the properties of a neural clock.

His logic was that the distance between two quite distant Purkinje cells can be measured by the time it takes for a signal to pass along the axons that run through the trees. But this also corresponds to a specific number of Purkinje cells. Count the number of trees separating Purkinje cells in an array and it is a readout of the time for a signal to pass between them. In Braitenberg's hypothesis, reading the position of collisions of inputs across the giant grid of Purkinje cells is like watching the constellation of intricate timing coincidences in all the signals the cerebellum receives. In other words, a Purkinje cell array converts time into space.

As what seemed like the perfect validation of this idea, in the mid-1960s, one animal was investigated with a cerebellum of such enormous size and crystalline precision in the arrangement of the Purkinje cell 'palisades' that it embodied a neural clock.[4] At first sight, the entire brain seemed to be pure cerebellum. This was the African elephant-nose fish (a member of the mormyrid family) first described scientifically by Walter Stendell and dubbed *Schnauzenorgane* in 1914.[5] Living in muddy water with limited visibility, these mormyrid fish evolved an ability to sense disturbances by using a self-generated, weak electric current in the water around them not only to feel their way through the gloom, but also to communicate with each other and court the opposite sex. The calculations required to compute an image of its murky aquatic world from electrical fields would require the millisecond comparisons of electrical disruption. The enormous size of the Purkinje cell arrays seemed perfect for the job. The mormyrid must, it seemed, rely on a hugely expanded number of precisely aligned Purkinje cells to interpret and interact with its world through a matrix of intricate timing calculations.

These first investigations of the mormyrid fish and Braitenberg's clock theories languished in the subsequent decades. In some ways, Braitenberg's thinking now seems rather quaint, superseded by techniques and ideas that look at brain function in a very different way. It also does not get close enough to giving predictable answers to experiments. It is more of a general feeling about architecture and form, and his sensitivity to the texture of brains is largely forgotten. And yet the perspectives of Purkinje, Golgi, Cajal and Braitenberg on form and function all speak to that compelling thought that, when looking at brain cells, this beauty is more than just convenience or accident . . . it must *mean* something.

Timing seems important for the cerebellum. Being able to dance, learn to play the piano or tap out a regular rhythm are all dependent on it working correctly. But maybe it is alertness to the surprises and mistakes that really lie at the heart of its millisecond-clock-hand Purkinje cells. Does this perhaps explain the less obvious part the cerebellum plays in our emotions and reasoning, telling us when something is not quite right or doesn't fit? It is down to the cerebellum that you are unable to tickle yourself. It knows what you are going to do before you do it – there are no surprises here. But logically, following this argument, it must also be the organ that allows you to be tickled and perhaps that is its purpose. The Purkinje cell isn't reading the world to help us kick a football better. It is calibrating our uncertainty and preparing us for the unexpected.

Cell 2

The pig barn and the retinal ganglion cell

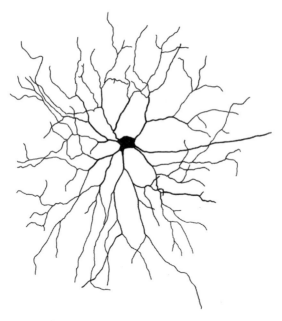

A single retinal ganglion cell – one of the larger of several varieties – drawn from multiple photographic negatives. The flattened dendritic trees of a whole population of these cells form a continuous mosaic, so that an even and complete sampling of the visual world is projected through the lens to the back of the eye.

I spent four years drawing one kind of cell in near darkness – the retinal ganglion cell. This is the cell that organises the basic grammar of our vision. It carries the visual message from our eyes to the brain, transmitting what our retina sees in its purest and most economical fashion. It is also a brain cell of near-crystalline dendritic symmetry, like the Purkinje cell, but arranged in a way that filters the visual world and generates pattern.

My retinal ganglion cell saga took place in an old pig barn reached by a short walk outdoors often in driving wind and rain. One part of this small shed, of indeterminate age, was sealed against daylight and set up by my father as an old-fashioned darkroom where he could print in black and white and, when feeling ambitious, colour. It also made an ideal space for me to take over to map the outlines of brain cells from photographs I had taken through the microscope back in the laboratory. Behind the wooden door of the barn, I slid strips of 35 mm celluloid negatives into an old Russian-made enlarger to project onto paper and trace in darkness.

There is a particular smell and touch to celluloid. Perhaps it is the lingering chemicals that are used to develop film; a sour, slightly tipsy odour that sticks to your hands. The more films I developed, the more liberal I became with the chemicals and the more the smell impregnated my life. In complete blackout, I became expert at measuring out thirty-six exposure lengths from a new tin of twenty metres of pristine, unexposed film. The only light was the unanticipated flash of blue that comes from the glue in Sellotape as it is peeled away – a discovery made while fixing the strips onto their spindles before they were rolled and packed into canisters that could be loaded into a camera.

Each film canister could capture images of maybe six brain cells, photographed at different levels of focus. If the cell was particularly large or wandered in and out of the optical depth of field it might take all thirty-six shots to photograph its structure. Once developed and dried, I fed the slivers of exposed negatives, six images at a time, through the metal lips of the enlarger and brought into focus small tendrils of shadow. I became used to the fact that although one's eyes rapidly adapt to the darkness, it might take thirty minutes to become completely sensitised. I also became obsessed with the quality of ink and maintaining my pens: cleaning, refilling and reconstructing their barrels, trying not to let the fine cylindrical nibs dry out.

The strips of monochrome, foggy with their sharp points of detail to be traced, seemed never-ending. Those four years melt away in my memory into the same few moments: the slow walk to the darkness of the pig barn, the sour smell of celluloid, the cold square of light.

I was searching for order, through the patterns in the crowd of neurons that laminate the back of the retina. Lying on top of the more familiar rods and cones that react directly to light are the cells that I spent four years drawing repeatedly – the ones that connect the eye to the brain: retinal ganglion cells. 'Retinal' because its body and its dendrites lie within the retina of the eye. 'Ganglion' refers to a collection of these bodies in a swelling, but, in this case, the bodies of retinal ganglion cells are scattered across the retina. The outputs of the cell – the axons – are bunched together at the start of the optic nerve, like the stems of a bouquet. This point on the retina, the 'blind spot' of your eye, is where the axons set out towards the brain in the optic nerve. This rush of inter-twined fibres leaving the eye through the toughened cable of the nerve are the sole bearers of all our visual information: our world, its inhabitants, colours, movements and the words you are reading now.

As is the case for most trainee scientists, this was a project that I had been given rather than chosen. It was up to me to find the fascination that would propel me on in the darkness. The more I drew and the more I read, the more extraordinary it began to seem that our world of vision is conjured from a retinal ganglion cell language that is patchy and counter-in-tuitive. Our construction of a perceptual world suddenly appeared to be a tremendous piece of theatre, engineered by our brains, to convince us that sensations are complete and reliable while concealing a script of hasty translations and omissions.

Do we all see colour in the same way? It is a frequent question that seems to get to the heart of a paradox. We can never truly experience the world through another being's senses. As I drew and reconstructed retinal ganglion cells, what I wanted to know was how it felt to see with the simplest of visual systems. What would be the shape of that world seen through the narrowest of perspectives?

This question had arisen in a chance, five-minute conversation with a legendary scientist, Richard Gregory (1923–2010), about plankton. Gregory had read something I had written about the snapshots and slices that I used to construct cells. He was bubbling with excitement over the similarities between my description and the visual world of a tiny marine invertebrate that he had studied in the 1950s in the marine biological laboratory in Naples. The experiments seemed a world away from my muddy pig barn, with its frequent rain showers and grey of a Devon winter. Gregory recounted his time at the Stazione Zoologica Anton Dohrn, which figures so heavily in the story of brain cells, and I felt a pang of envy of the warmth of the Mediterranean sun. I had a fantasy of him thirty years previously, in a small boat, out for the day to catch specimens for the lab, and then pulling hard for the shore, returning to a fantastic meal and a bottle of red wine overlooking a glittering bay. No doubt the reality was somewhat different, but the sun-infused story stuck with me and I searched out his account of a curious eye he had found, published in the magazine *Nature* in the 1960s.

Gregory's quarry had been a copepod called *Copilia quadrata*, one of the myriad of small planktonic creatures, and his fascination stemmed from its visual system – the simplest arrangement that he could imagine for reconstructing a visual world. He described a creature whose 'eyes' are nothing more than two detector cells that scanned across the visual world like the beam in a cathode ray tube found in the first television. Using just a rapid horizontal sweep of its submarine world, 200 metres below the surface, *Copilia* could hunt and navigate its environment.[6] This is vision stripped back to its simplest form. And yet, with only two scanning sensors, the copepod builds up a picture of the world that is sufficient – enough to thrive. At great depths in the Bay of Naples, the creature detects flecks of reflected light, collected by two tubes capped by optical lenses. At the other end of each tube, the single biological light detector responds when a photon is caught and focused by the lens onto five sensing cells that detect a single picture element or pixel.[7] The tubes scan horizontally, both moving out slowly to the edges of what is a field of vision and springing back to 'looking' dead ahead, moving through a single narrow line. They don't look up, they don't focus, they scan.

I wondered what the world looked like for *Copilia*. I can take a guess that any bright spot moving horizontally at the same speed as the pivoting tubes into a position directly ahead would give a sustained stimulus to its 'eyes'. Anything moving in the opposite direction, away from the animal, would barely be detected – almost invisible. This would be a world shaped by horizontal movements. Was it enough information for the miniature animal to grab its food or possibly to escape? The limitations of two, single light detectors on pivots, seeing the narrowest of slices of possibilities, seem obvious. Its picture of the world was enough for *Copilia* but huge swathes of visual information were ignored. But, it then seemed to me, *Copilia* sees none of these limitations. Its visual world is complete and untroubling and, in that fundamentally important sense, it is exactly the same as ours.

Our visual detectors are also limited. The picture they give us of the world is fragmentary and yet seems to us complete and satisfactory – marvellous in fact. The biggest and most important job of the visual system is to take the fragmentary channels of information, routed through retinal ganglion cells, and convince us that what we see is, like a neural version of Voltaire's Professor Pangloss, the best of all possible worlds.

What differs in our visual world from that of plankton is the dimensions of information that we process. Whereas *Copilia* has two channels that survey a thin strip of an underwater world, we have millions of channels fixed in our retina, and our whole eye is moved to follow objects that interest or startle us. Each of these millions of channels is conveyed by a retinal ganglion cell; each retinal ganglion cell carries a message about the changing patterns of light in a single pixel. Where *Copilia* has two parallel streams of information from scanners, we have many, sitting side by side in a mosaic that tiles the back of our eyes.

To make sense of the patterns of light falling onto the retina, there is not just a single mosaic, but multiple layers of retinal ganglion cells, each containing its own distinct style of dendritic tree. Retinal ganglion cells come in different forms, from dense shrubby tangled rose bushes to languid, elegant branching trees that spread gracefully across the retina. They all send long axons through the optic nerve to the brain. All transmit an interpretation of the light patterns that fall on the retina, either by reading what our rods and cones are saying or, in a small minority of cases, directly responding to light. These different types of retinal ganglion cells, each population completely tiling the retina, embody the essence of how we see.

The smaller denser cells have intricately branched dendrites that seem to greedily grasp the contacts with rods and cones; the largest have a more expansive dendritic tree that stretches out like the fractal fingers of lightning. And between these two extremes a myriad of branching shapes and flattened dendrites are flat and laid out in a mosaic across the retina. My job as a student was to uncover these forms and one by one, painfully slowly, I collected different types of retinal ganglion cell dendrites, cataloguing the differences in how they fanned out from the cell body.

What I was piecing together, sitting in the pig barn, was only a fragmentary contribution to an understanding of the visual world whose logic was taking shape from the work of hundreds of different scientists. The picture emerging from all these studies was that it seemed most likely that a single type of retinal ganglion cell would make a mosaic with only its own kind. The mosaics of each type would then be layered on top of each other, one after the other, building up laminae that were, in effect, different kinds of filters of the visual world. The smallest cells responded slowly to changing light patterns, but because their mosaic was dense and made up of tiny dendritic trees, the world they communicated was a sharply etched picture with separate channels for blue, green and red light. Retinal ganglion cells with the largest dendritic trees would be spaced more generously with a mosaic of larger tiles. Their world was consequently a blur made of giant pixels in monochrome, but one that responded quickly to change. We rely on the small cells for a detailed picture of the world in colour. The information from larger cells alerts our brains to events and drives our attention. And in between, a world of different retinal ganglion cells gives a translation of the visual scene in a constellation of different ways.

Juxtaposing this picture of how our visual machinery works with Richard Gregory's Neapolitan creature, the massive gulf in sophistication from human to plankton seemed obvious. Whereas *Copilia* scans a small segment of the visual world sequentially, our retina samples the whole scene simultaneously with overlapping mosaics of retinal ganglion cells extracting different kinds of information from the photoreceptors that respond to light. However, just like *Copilia*, our brains are forced to make up a story out of information that, despite all the elaborate retinal ganglion cell types, is a collection of fragments.

For a start, retinal ganglion cells only send signals about change in light intensity. If we could stabilise the pattern of light falling on our rods and cones, the retinal ganglion cells that listen only for change would essentially fall asleep. Our eyes would fall silent even as our brains maintain a picture, at least for a while, like a frozen frame in a film.

Our visual world is a meticulously constructed model and all our eyes serve to do is tweak and mould with splashes of new information relayed by retinal ganglion cells.

Not only do our retinal ganglion cells only bother to tell us about change, but only the most densely packed mosaics at the fovea of the retina are used to paint a detailed picture of the world. At the fovea (the point on the retina where the sharpest visual information is collected), retinal ganglion cells are crowded into a dense huddle. Their dendritic trees are tiny, each sampling a miniature pixel-width of vision: the more pixels, the more detail is captured.

Our eyes are constantly moving to direct the fovea to where the action is. Speedy signals from the large retinal ganglion cells outside the fovea alert our brain to changes around us, driving our six eye muscles to reorientate our gaze. Vision is an active and relentless search to update our model of the world. Whereas *Copilia* scans without an obvious goal, our eyes swivel and focus driven by an unconscious need to attend to every change in the outside world.

Nothing perhaps shows the construction and outright trickery more clearly than the huge holes in our vision that we completely cover over at our 'blind spot' in each eye. This is the optic disc – a part of the retina where there is no space for photoreceptors, pushed aside by retinal ganglion cells' axons which funnel out of the retina alongside blood vessels. It leaves a surprisingly huge visual hole, which is painted over by the brain but which can be uncovered by playing with two shapes and a piece of paper.

You can reveal your own blind spot quite easily. It is a simple test – and maybe one you have done before. On a piece of paper, draw a cross and a circle about ten centimetres apart. Close one eye and with the open eye fix your focus on the symbol closest to your nose. Now, move the paper away from your face and then bring it closer again. When the page is about thirty centimetres from your eye, the symbol that you are not focusing on – the one to the outer edge of your visual field – will disappear.

This is dramatic and surprising. But, for me, the truly exciting part of this remarkable trick is when you draw the same symbols on a piece of text such as an old newspaper. Try this again for yourself and, as before, the symbol that you are not focusing on (away from your nose) will disappear. However, this time the text, underneath the circle or cross that you have drawn, remains. Our brain completes the picture for us, filling in the hole with the most plausible background – text, colour, the street outside or a face whose completeness we only think we see. We never notice objects disappearing as they pass across the blind spot. It is only by forcing our attention in this way that we can glimpse it. The brain will never allow us to see our partial blindness.

Because information to the brain is rationed by the retinal ganglion cells, the brain becomes susceptible to optical illusion and optical ambiguity. But it is also quicker to respond and because it is working with a model it can jump ahead to anticipate. We recognise and name at the same time as we see. The parts of our brain that are tuned to faces, for example, are poised to leap into action. When this patch of neurons involved in face recognition is damaged, deep in the cerebral cortex, we are sometimes unable to compensate; face blindness (prosopagnosia) is a difficult handicap to work round. But at the level of the retinal ganglion cell's message, our visual machinery is expert at filling in the gaps. Vision is a story told by the cortex about a world constructed from the fragments transmitted by retinal ganglion cells.

What would it be like if vision was not a story but a literal translation of signals from a retinal ganglion cell? What if we saw the gaps and the blind spots, and were constantly aware of the blurriness at the edge of our visual fields? Or what if we, disturbingly, detected that colour arrives in the brain more slowly than movement? Our world would be jarring, unsettling and uncertain; to me, it seems that the work of vision is to patch up the holes left by the cells that I sat drawing in the pig barn. I felt sure that a central job of any brain is to make sure this never happens. So although from the outside we can see the deficiencies of Richard Gregory's *Copilia*, I am certain that *Copilia*, suspended in the deep blue in the Bay of Naples, with only its two retinal ganglion cells, feels just as reassured and certain as we are that it is seeing the best of all possible visual worlds.

Cell 3

The astrocyte and neural glue

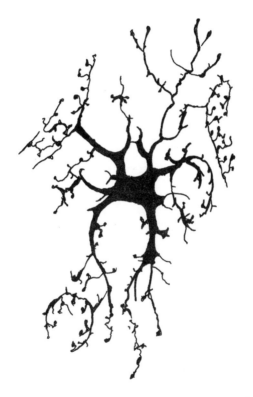

Small and delicate astrocytes do not carry messages. Instead, they maintain the environment within the brain. The shape of their arms, or 'processes', describe the ghostly form of an invisible neuronal cell body and microscopic blood vessels.

No brain cell is more than a few cells' width away from a supply of oxygen. The brain is full of blood and about one fifth of all the circulating oxygen that is carried by red blood cells is needed to keep our brain cells working. The major arteries run over the surface of the brain and spinal cord, but millions of smaller vessels penetrate beneath its surface, dividing again and again to make a continuous mesh of microscopic blood-filled capillaries. And wrapped around the miniature capillaries are astrocytes. Complex, branching, beautiful, intricate, exploding like starbursts inside our heads.

Astrocytes are small and delicately strung between blood vessels and neural brain cells. The distinction between neural and non-neural is important. Non-neural brain cells, like the astrocyte, have always been recognised as something outside the communication channels in the brain that make sense of the world and control our actions. The non-neural brain cells are a massive and somewhat mysterious crowd that clean up after the neurons, hold the fabric of the brain itself together and have generally lived in the shadows of their larger and more showy cousins.

The astrocyte clings to the blood supply of the brain and is found everywhere that you look. You only really get a sense of the density of the matted capillary mesh of blood vessels when everything else is, literally, dissolved away. When I first studied biology as an undergraduate, I noticed that, tucked away on top of the wooden bookcases lining the corridor of the university department, there was an eerie collection of animal shapes, seemingly sculpted in blue and red threads. These were the blood supplies of entire animals, extracted by material science and chemistry, intact from the bodies of their former hosts. Generations of final-year students had made these casts as their laboratory projects – the red and blue meshes once arteries and veins of deceased cats, rats or ferrets.

Each cast was the product of corrosion. Arteries and veins had been injected with methyl methacrylate, which filled the branching network to its finest tips and then set hard. The muscle, fat and bone were then dissolved away to leave a perfect model of the host – a ghost in blood.

Corrosion casting is an ancient technique, dating back to the seventeenth century when closely guarded recipes that combined wax, clay, paraffin, vermillion, bismuth or mercury were used by scientists such as Robert Boyle to probe the anatomy of blood.[8, 9] Newer methods led to finer and finer details being revealed down to the levels seen only, in modern techniques, by a microscope. And it is here that the richness of the network of vessels in the brain becomes clear. When a corrosion cast is made of the delicate blood-filled channels permeating throughout the brain, it is a solid sponge of entwined tubes. Microcapillaries penetrate every cranny and, although invisible to the corrosion cast, every surface of each vessel is tiled by the miniature protrusions of a vast population of astrocytes.

At the beginning of the story of the brain and its cells, the black reaction of Camillo Golgi set up the great divide between nerve cells, which made connections that must underlie thought, and a second population of intricate, non-neural forms, which emerged, ornate and beautiful, from a substance that had forty years earlier been called the neuroglia – neural glue.

The word neuro-glia was first used by Rudolf Virchow[i] (1821–1902) in 1856, to describe what sat between the tangled fibres of the brain: an amorphous material, a nerve putty (*nervenkitt*) that held the tissue together.[10] To Virchow's eyes, the space seemed to be full of the broken pieces of cells – a multitude of cell nuclei but nothing more, floating in a gel.

With the later arrival of Golgi's black reaction, it suddenly became clear that the nuclei in the gel were not abandoned remnants, nor the multinucleate fungus-like intrusions, but formed the tiny heart of a menagerie of sometimes miniature cells, some of which, like the astrocyte, were in every way as complex and intricately branched as a neuron. However, the label of glue, putty or gel, stuck. The various and varied populations, astrocytes included, were grouped together as glue or 'glia'.

Why was it so obvious that glia were different from neurons? Something about the way they thread their way between other cells, or stretch out as if to hold tissue together and cling to microscopic blood vessels spoke of structure and support. The cascading tiers of crenulations in the stately Bergmann glia in the cerebellum and the pine-tree-like rows of Müller cells in the retina were architectural buttresses that seemed to hold the brain together. Astrocytes were the closest to neurons in the way they branched and spread outwards from a cell body, but if you look closely at the tips of each you find a blood vessel.

When Santiago Ramón y Cajal first drew astrocytes, they appeared to him to be tiny, delicate insulators forming a layer sandwiched between the nerve cell and its blood supply. He believed that the millions of astrocytes spread through the brain were best thought of as a single gland, scattered cells acting as a collective organ. He imagined it regulating the amount of blood reaching brain cells, supplying more to regions that were particularly active.[11]

One thing that also stood out was just how many more astrocytes were present in the human brain than in the brains of other animals. The hugely expanded brain volume in man is not due to an increase in the number of nerve cells but perhaps only to the number of astrocytes. One answer to why this might be is found in sleep.

To understand why, we have to go back to one of the other discoveries made by Rudolf Virchow while exploring the spaces in the brain. Virchow seemed to have a gift for looking between the lines of anatomy and into the gaps that others had ignored. As he scanned the microscopic blood vessels threading their way between the large and small nuclei of neural and non-neural cells, he noticed that the vessels appeared to have an extra 'skin'. Blood vessels sat inside a thin outer glove and between these was a very fine but distinct gap. Virchow and the French anatomist Charles-Phillipe Robin gave their names jointly to the Virchow–Robin space. This is the outer sleeve to which the thickened club-like endings of the branching arms of astrocytes lock. They are not sampling blood as first supposed. Instead, the vanishingly small gap between the blood and astroglia is part of a shadow circulatory system, unique to the brain, of a thin, watery liquid, cerebrospinal fluid, conveyed by Virchow–Robin spaces to every recess that can be reached by blood.

Cerebrospinal fluid is closely associated with the large cavities that sit at the heart of the brain, called ventricles. The first anatomists, dissecting the soft, collapsing, unpreserved brains of animals and man, noticed seemingly empty chambers at the heart of the brain. The existence of chambers had excited a range of ideas in the intervening millennia about what they contained – how they might be a storage for the essential animal spirit that controlled the body. For many centuries, they were seen as the engine of the brain's function. Galen, who was a doctor to both gladiators and emperors in ancient Rome, and whose work shaped medieval medicine, saw them as a reservoir of a psychological energy, secreted by the brain. This was central to his theory that it was the brain and not the heart that controlled the body.

The first mention of a liquid inside the brain dates back to an Egyptian papyrus from 3000–2500 BC, but it was not until 1536 that it was described again with any certainty, by Nicolo Massa. It was given the name cerebrospinal fluid by François Magendie (1783–1855) in 1828, who discovered that the chambers were connected by channels, and also to the surface of the brain by the eponymous foramen of Magendie.[ii] Magendie's cerebrospinal fluid is what doctors extract in a spinal tap, when a needle is carefully inserted into the space between vertebrae. Because the ventricles of the brain and the canal at the centre of the spinal cord are continuous, what takes place in the brain can be read at the spinal cord by changes in the half a litre of cerebrospinal fluid that is made each day.

Magendie also noticed that the fluid pulses in time with

breathing. These fluxes pump the liquid out onto the surface of the brain where it is trapped underneath layers of membranes called the meninges.[12] Within this membrane-lined space, filled with cerebrospinal fluid, sit the major arteries that course over the surface of the brain and send tiny branches deep between the neurons. And on the outside of these vessels, tracking along inside the narrowest gap of the Virchow–Robin space, cerebrospinal fluid flows deep into the brain to feed the network of astrocytes.

The role of this fluid was believed at first to be as a drain for waste metabolites and as a supporting cushion against the shocks and collisions of bony skull and vertebrae that surround our brain and spinal cord. From the 1920s through to the 1970s, it was considered so dispensable that it could be sucked out of the base of the spinal cord and replaced with helium or air. In an agonising procedure, patients were then rotated to move the air about the internal cavities of the brain before an X-ray was performed. A gas-filled cavity shows up on an X-ray in a way that cerebrospinal fluid, with almost an identical specific density to brain tissue, does not. Ventriculography allowed radiographers to gauge the internal structure of ventricles that would otherwise be impenetrable to the X-ray machine. Once drained for the procedure, the ventricles simply filled again with fluid over the course of a day.

Relegating the ventricles to subsidiary structures made it possible to overlook a vital function for cerebrospinal fluid as the reservoir for a nightly irrigation choreographed by astrocytes. As we dream, the astrocytes embark on the job of brain washing – sluicing the cell spaces of all the rubbish that has accumulated during the day. The tips of the astrocyte arms draw the water from the cerebrospinal fluid in the narrow

Virchow–Robin spaces around micro-arteries and wash the accumulated debris and proteins away.[13] This includes the harmful protein amyloid beta, long associated with Alzheimer's disease. During sleep or induced sleep by anaesthesia, the fluid between brain cells increases by more than half. The outflows for our brain wash are the Virchow–Robin spaces surrounding veins. The purification complete, we wake.

How exactly astrocytes regulate blood flow and brain washing is yet to be discovered. There is something compelling about the image of this network of tiny cells, like a sponge, deeply integrated between our neurons and our blood supply, acting as a single organ of protection. This was Cajal's idea when he first drew the tiny starbursts of astrocytes and it is now perhaps made more compelling by an understanding of how they bathe our brain cells as we sleep. Is there something special about the human brain that requires so many more astrocytes than any other animal? Perhaps it is the intensity of our thoughts, the resources we use and the daily build-up of their by-products, rather than simply the number of our neurons, that say something about what it is to have a human brain.

As we grow old, something happens to the spaces that astrocytes guard. Just as our skin wrinkles and droops, the Virchow–Robin gaps between the blood vessel and astrocytes begin to sag and dilate. Cerebrospinal fluid starts to push inwards from the surface of the brain, widening the normally tight spaces around the capillaries, pushing the astrocytes away from the blood cells just a few thousandths of a millimetre away. It is unclear why this happens. But perhaps astrocytes, suspended between the neurons and their blood supply, washing the brain night after night, have had enough.

Rather than drawing out the liquid they need to rinse out the gaps between neurons, the water channels (aquaporins) at the tips of their branches perhaps begin to shut down. Imperceptibly at first, but far too early in some who suffer dementia, the widening of the Virchow–Robin space creeps along the microscopic vessels that weave between the brain cells. The flow of fluid into the brain becomes more sluggish and the cocoon of astrocytes that protects and nourishes our vast population of neurons is gently eased back, deeper into the recesses of the brain.

Cell 4

The sensory cell, Cajal's mistake and Freud's throwback

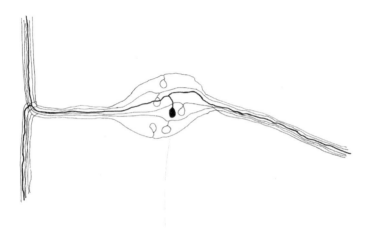

The sensory cells receive signals from an axon that stretches from the body (up) and send information about pain, touch, pressure, heat, cold etc. to the central nervous system (down). The naked cell body is clustered with other, mute neighbours (outlined) within a ganglion. A series of ganglia run up and down the spine where nerves enter the cord.

Not all brain cells are spectacular to look at. With the stripped-back elegance of Bauhaus furniture, the sensory cell is a minimalist neuron. It links our skin and muscles to our central nervous system, telling us when we are stroked or warning us when we touch something hot or overstretch a limb. Although it will never make the front cover of a textbook, or the inside pages of a celebration of neuroanatomical art, there is something necessarily visually compelling in its simplicity. It has an important part in the story of the brain in revealing the language of how cells communicate. Its simple structure was a cause of confusion and debate, but ultimately opened a door to ideas about how brain cells evolved and perhaps even shaped Freud's thinking on how our minds retain ancestral impulses and urges.

We have long known where these brain cells insert themselves between the nervous system and our body. Long axons stretch from the spinal cord to muscles and skin and, in a most particular way, their cell bodies huddle close together in nodules called ganglia that button their way up the outside of the spinal cord and hindbrain. They are unique in lacking any form of dendrite – the elaborate and extravagant flourishes that give cells like the Purkinje neuron their character and function. The ganglion houses a sheltering cluster of naked, sensory cell bodies. Stretching in both directions, long axons push along nerves both to receive signals from and direct them to the spinal cord and brain.

All the sensory neuron cell bodies of the nerve, which together lay down a cable of wiring, are cloistered into the tightly bound space of the ganglion. They are a self-contained annexe to the central nervous system – peripheral, out of reach with the myriads of brain cells that jam the spinal cord and the brain. And with no dendrites, sensory cell bodies have no means of talking to each other. They sit side by side, each passing on their own piece of the message, unable to share a conversation: a monastic community, blind to their neighbours and uninterested in the information that they traffic. In contrast to all other brain cells, their cell body makes no attempt to change or interpret the signals they spend their lives relaying – it simply watches the information flow by.

The simple structure of these sensory neurons means they are rarely depicted as anything more than a simple symbol on a circuit diagram of a reflex. Consequently, as I learned the basics of neuroscience at school, I never questioned that peculiar simplicity that popped up time and again in diagrams of how reflexes work. The axon was an unbranching line that stretched out from the body to the central nervous system. Somewhere close to the spinal cord, a small ball – a cell body – would sit on top of a tiny branch sticking out from the axon. The T-shape of its structure is instantly recognisable in any textbook drawing but rarely a cause for curiosity.

*   *   *

However, sensory neurons were the first brain cells to give a clue to the nature of messages that travel through to the brain – the small packets of electricity that light up connections with a rapid sputtering of activity, the hum of the wiring. Although Galvani had shown in the 1700s that electricity would cause a frog muscle to twitch, the role of electricity or whether indeed it was used by nerves was still unclear at the end of the 1800s.

A new technology was needed to listen in to the tiny signals passed between brain cells The solution came from the introduction of the valve amplifier into the laboratory. Sitting inside a sealed glass tube, a heated wire fired electrons across a vacuum in a stream that could be halted or vastly accelerated by the tiniest of signals. The fluctuations in the tiny signal could now be used to control sound, a column of mercury or the movement of needle: amplifiers became a crucial multi-purpose tool. Valves were replaced by semiconductors but the amplifier itself never disappeared. And so, in front of my own microscope, sitting in darkness, even though I rarely recorded the activities of neurons, an amplifier helped me to navigate between their densely packed cell bodies with the tip of a glass tube.

To fill a brain cell with a brightly fluorescent yellow dye, you have to sit and listen. The dye sits in a glass pipette with a sharp point so fine it's invisible to the naked eye. Even though you can't see when the sharpened glass tube touches the surface of a cell, you can hear it. The fluid-filled microscopic tip is linked to an amplifier via a thin sliver of silver wire pushed down the open, blunt end of the glass and in turn to a voltage control oscillator (VCO), which turns electrical signals to audible tones.

I'm trying to hear my way towards a cell. At the far end of my glass tube, the tip had been heated up and then pulled to a fine tip through which the dye would be injected. But as this tip pushes against the boundaries of a cell, the free flow of ions is sealed off and they pile up; the electrical resistance shoots up and the pitch of my VCO falls to a bass hum. As I push the dye-filled glass towards a neuron under the microscope, I listen to the signal through an amplifier. The pitch suddenly dips. I want to flood the cell with dye, break the obstruction and rip a hole in the fragile membrane that surrounds the cell body. A single tap to the table, a stamp of my foot on the floor – anything to create the smallest vibration is enough to push the sharpened tip of glass into the cell body. Dye pours in and the neuron begins to fill with dazzling yellow.

Sitting alongside my new microscope are my discrete, modern digital amplifiers, packed into their convenient tower of racks. And behind those, high up on a shelf or tucked into a corner, are the bulky, grey metal-cased laboratory electronics of another age. Valve amplifiers with the name ADRIAN inked across them, in bold capitals. It's almost child-like, partly because it appears to be someone's first name. It wasn't until much later that I realised that these were artefacts of fundamental discovery in neuroscience, handed down like family heirlooms from supervisor to student. This was their fourth generation of inheritance and the original owner was a pioneer of electrical recording in the brain: Lord Edgar Adrian, my supervisor's supervisor's supervisor's supervisor – my research great-great-grandfather.

The amplifiers that first made the sound of nerve cells audible were invented at the start of the twentieth century and began making their appearance in laboratories in the early 1920s.

Edgar Adrian (1889–1977) was a young First World War veteran who seized on this state-of-the-art technology, recognising the possibilities to build on the pre-war studies that he had conducted with his scientific mentor, Keith Lucas (1879–1916). Their research had been housed in a dark, smelly and often flooded cellar housing a cottage industry of experimentation. It was here that Lucas made a crucial discovery about the nature of electrical activity of nerves. Like Galvani before him, Lucas used frog muscle to study the role of electricity in movement. He found that nerve impulses that controlled muscles were 'all or nothing'.[14] A stimulus had to reach a certain threshold to cause a muscle to contract and stronger contractions were the result of more units of muscle being activated. This hinted that nerve cells might talk to other cells using packets of information: more like a morse code than music. However, the nature of this language remained elusive without a means of listening directly to what cells were saying.

It was at this point that the First World War interrupted their work. When Edgar Adrian returned to Cambridge, still only in his twenties, it was without his closest collaborator. Adrian had spent most of the previous four years treating patients with shell shock in Aldershot; Keith Lucas, who had volunteered for the Royal Flying Corps, had died in a mid-air collision.

Determined to continue his friend's research into how brain cells talked to each other, Adrian found a department that had been radically transformed from its former damp subterranean nooks into a gleaming research unit. He set out to understand whether the signals in sensory nerves – taking information from the body to the brain – were working in a similar way to Lucas' signals that controlled muscles. He knew that when muscles were stretched, they alerted the spinal cord using sensory neurons. Were the signals they transmitted the small packets of morse code that Lucas had hypothesised?

Adrian bought a newly perfected valve amplifier, capable of taking a fluctuation of millivolts and expanding it to a voltage that could be translated into a visible signal. He connected the amplifier to an electrometer which, like a thermometer, registered signals in the movement of a thin column of mercury housed in glass. The mercury column would twitch up and down following a change in voltage. All that was required was to attach one end of the wire to a nerve and the other to the amplified input and any electrical signal would be registered by the dancing thread of silver.

But the equipment was temperamental, and Adrian tried successively simpler configurations to reduce the number of variable factors that seemed to be confounding his experiments. However he attached the wires to a piece of dissected frog muscle, all he saw was 'noisy' signal – a random fluttering of mercury column that never settled. He began to despair of this new temperamental technology.

After hours of fiddling, checking for loose connections and retracing his steps in rebuilding his apparatus, Adrian suddenly realised that the chatter had a pattern, and that the pattern changed whenever he inadvertently allowed the muscle to touch the glass plate over which it was suspended. If he lifted the glass plate or lowered the muscle, the noise stopped. When the muscle fragment was hanging in an experimental chamber over its glass plate unsupported, it was shouting its discomfort through rapid volleys of signals from stretch receptors. Adrian had seen in the chorus of sensory neurons what no one had before: the language of brain cells.

66

For Edgar Adrian it was a moment that made him pause to reflect on the random nature of discoveries. All the ingenuity and technology that had made the moment possible still did not lead to the moment of revelation without the intervention of chance. It was everything, he wrote, that he could wish for: 'it didn't involve any particular hard work or any particular intelligence', just a combination of circumstance, tinkering and accident.[i, 15]

What Adrian had discovered were the signals of sensory cells that respond to stretching a muscle – the impulses that tell our knee to jerk upwards when tapped with a hammer. But different sensory cells can give different kinds of information about what is happening in our bodies or on our skin depending on the proteins embedded at their tips. These proteins form tiny holes or channels into nerve endings that can open or close to let ions into the tips of sensory cells. Some open when compressed: when we touch or are touched. Some open when heated or when cooled. Any one of these sensations comes down to the changing shape of microscopic proteins and regulating a rush of ions that launches an impulse along a nerve fibre.

The receptors explain how our perceptions are sometimes clustered together in ways that make sense to us but have no objective logic. The receptor that contorts itself to pour ions into a nerve ending when we put chilli pepper in our mouth is the same that responds to high temperatures on our skin. We call both sensations 'heat'. An evolutionary tweak in its structure and careful placement on the nerve endings on the lips and nose of vampire bats allows them to detect the heat in a sweet spot for drawing blood as they swoop over the skin of their prey.

67

When things go wrong in the same nerve in humans, a similar super-sensitisation causes the most painful diseases we can suffer. It results in an absolute horror of being touched, for fear of triggering excruciating agony. 'Trigeminal neuralgia' can be traced down the centuries as tic douloureux[ii] and Fothergill's disease,[16] in the writings of the philosopher and physician John Locke,[17] and as far back to Avicenna and Galen in Roman times.

The causes are still unknown but somehow the primary sensory neurons of the trigeminal ganglion abandon their orderly and faithful transmission of signals and instead yell to be heard. Imagine that neurons have a personality. Here are the disenfranchised cell bodies of the sensory neuron, so often overlooked, considered unglamorous, but central to the story of the neuron, as we learn from Edgar Adrian's discovery. It's easy to imagine they may have seized the opportunity that neuralgia afforded to step out from the shadows and shout.

The shape of a primary sensory cell is truly unipolar – its cell body a functional dead end. Nothing passes through it and it plays no role in shaping how information is transmitted. However, this is not how things began in the life of a sensory neuron. In younger cells, the cell body sits squarely between a dendrite and an axon. Young sensory neurons are not unipolar but bipolar. The primary sensory neuron starts as a cell body with, on one side, a single, very long dendrite extending to a receptor in the body and, on the other side, an axon sending information into the spinal cord or brain. The cell resembles a string with a single bead threaded onto it. At some point the cell body is shoved out of the way, onto

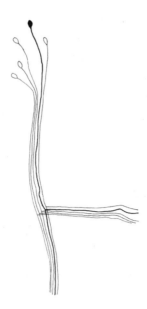

The only sensory neurons buried in the brain form the scattered components of the mesencephalic trigeminal nucleus. One arm (to the right) receives information about bite pressure from teeth and relays it down into the hindbrain.

its pedicle, and it is relieved of any opportunity to shape the function of the cell.[iii]

The small pedicle within the ganglion is always short. Perhaps its length depends on how much crowding there is within the ganglion; the reasons are unknown. However, there is one sensory cell where the pedicle is extremely long – too long to be the outcome of some displacement. Too long for the pedicle to have originated in the same way as other sensory neurons. And furthermore, this 'mesencephalic trigeminal' primary sensory neuron sits inside the brain: the only adult sensory neuron in vertebrates to do so.

Its shape, position and questions about its function weave a history of controversy. A tale of how the smallest nuances in form can obsess generations of neuroscientists, dividing them into two camps. And a tale that weaves together stories of evolution with the origins of psychoanalysis.

However, for me, one of this cell's startling features is that it seems to have confused and tricked Santiago Ramón y Cajal. I had bought a copy of his *Structure of the Nervous System* (a second edition with French text produced in 1911), paying a month's salary for it. The beauty of the images, some in two colours, some simply in black or a pale blue ink were worth the cost that, embarrassed, I kept to myself. It's the kind of book you can browse; each image is beautiful, hand-drawn by Cajal rather than a team of draughtsmen. But on one page something was not quite right. Cajal's description of this single brain cell seemed at odds with the accepted function of the mesencephalic trigeminal neuron as a sensory cell. I had to pause and read back, trying to translate the French in different ways. There was no doubting that he had made a mistake.

Remember that Cajal was there at the start of the story of the brain cell and perhaps was the central protagonist in the new neuroscience. By sticking to his interpretation of function by form he was, to my eyes, infallible. He had remarkable success in making bold statements about form and function that remain as true today as they were in the late nineteenth century. I had stumbled across what seemed to be an error.

I was primed to dig a little deeper because I had accidentally encountered this cell type myself, in the lab, trying to study something quite different. I was injecting a bright red fluorescent carbocyanine dye into the trigeminal nerve of a chicken embryo – the same nerve that triggers neuralgia in humans. Carbocyanine dyes dissolve into the lipids of cell membrane and rapidly diffuse over the entire surface of anything they touch. Carefully placing a crystal or solution of the bright scarlet dye allowed me to trace any axon leaving the brain back to its source.

The only axons that left the brain, as far as I was aware of at the time, were cells that controlled muscle movements: motor neurons. The trigeminal nerve has many of these, whose cell bodies I expected to see close to where the nerve exited the brain. However, far away from the point where my dye was injected into an embryonic chick, I could see a cluster of cell bodies, their axons clearly exiting through the nerve, but with unmistakeable, unipolar cell bodies deeply embedded in the distant midbrain. There were no dendrites. These were cells with T-shaped branching axons – sensory cells but with an extraordinarily long pedicle.

It did not take long to work out the cells in my photograph, looking like the arcs of unexploded fireworks; shooting into the sky were the mesencephalic trigeminal neurons. It would turn out, to my surprise, that these seemingly insignificant populations of sensory neurons had been at the centre of the long history of controversy, discussion and debate.

These were also the cells that had fooled Cajal. Although he puzzled at their unusual similarity to a sensory neuron, the trajectory of the axons, entwined with other motor outputs, and the position of their cell bodies – not huddled in a ganglion but scattered in the midbrain – meant that he could not believe they were anything but motor neurons.

This was the logic that governed his interpretation of the neuron information flow. Their specific trajectory towards the jaw led him to speculate that these were the brain cells that controlled chewing.[iv]

For Cajal the interpretation was obvious but ultimately proved incorrect. And at the time, it met with opposition from a small band of younger scientists, working with the species that Cajal had to some extent ignored: aquatic vertebrates, amphibians and reptiles.[v] A new journal, the *Journal of Comparative Neurology and Psychology*, was dedicated to reporting their observations, edited by Judson Herrick, who had written a book on the brain of the tiger salamander. The journal gathered the ideas and observations of biologists who were fascinated by the variation of structure between animal brains and how it might have evolved.

One of this new breed of comparative neuroanatomists was J. B. Johnston (1868–1939) from Ohio, who turned his attention to the mesencephalic trigeminal neuron and the key issue of which way information flowed within its unipolar, T-shaped form.[vi, 18] Johnston saw neuroanatomy through the new lens of evolution, a burgeoning idea at the time. He was particularly interested in species whose evolutionary ancestors were close to or came just before the emergence of backboned fish.

In species like the lancelet, a small arrow-shaped marine creature, halfway between a vertebrate and an invertebrate, the normal logic of sensory cells is reversed. Sensory cell bodies sit centrally and send their axons outwards. And when Johnston looked at the larvae of several fish species, he saw more of these kinds of primitive sensory cells. Like primary sensory cells, they also had large cell bodies without dendrites. He found them relaying the sensation of touch on the skin of a baby fish and again in tadpoles of amphibians. But only in jawless fish did they persist. In other vertebrates, the familiar unipolar, primary sensory neurons sitting within ganglia outside the central nervous system took over this job as the animal developed. In animals that had made the transition to land, the primitive sensory system had disappeared altogether.

In other words, there seemed to be a more ancient, sensory system with cell bodies in the brain, just like the mesencephalic trigeminal neurons, that gradually disappeared in the evolution of increasingly sophisticated animals. With these observations in mind, it seemed easy to imagine that the mesencephalic trigeminal neuron could itself be a sensory cell. Rather than controlling chewing as Cajal believed, the mesencephalic trigeminal neurons do the exact opposite: they relay the sensation of mastication to the brain. Specifically, their nerve endings are embedded in the pulp of the tooth sense pressure when we bite.

The need for sensation, in the least tactile of the structures on the surface of our body, seems to be an essential enabler of one of the most important evolutionary steps taken by vertebrates – the emergence of a jaw. The most primitive vertebrates, the ones closest to our common ancestors, do not possess jaws but instead have tentacles that surround a circular opening at the front end of their body. These are lampreys and hagfish, the majority of which retain an ancient micro-predatory lifestyle feeding off the bodies of larger fish to which they attach with their circular mouths.

The innovation of a jaw allowed vertebrates to be far more ambitious in the food that they could gather, moving from micro- to macro-predatory creatures. However, they also needed a sensor on their teeth to tell them how hard to bite

73

and when to stop biting. The ancestor of the mesencephalic trigeminal neuron was a sensory cell in the brain of jawless fish, recruited to this essential task and fixed ever since. The mesencephalic trigeminal neuron is the brain cell that allowed us to bite and chew – something that lamprey and the hagfish cannot do.

The question of the form of these cells set up battle lines in the neuroanatomical community. This was not just a question about the status of a peculiar and small population of brain cells, it was a question that niggled at the fundamental assumptions that Cajal had made about the shape, the topology, of brain cells. Famous names lined up with or against Johnston. Siding with Cajal were Wallenberg, Kolliker, Van Gehuchten, Held – each of them distinguished neuroscientists with structures in the brain that still bear their names. Kolliker stated that Johnston's interpretation would be an 'impossibility'. Others such as Meynert (the first to spot the mesencephalic trigeminal neuron) and Florence Sabine, a rare female pioneer of neuroscience in the early 1900s and a medical school contemporary of Gertrude Stein, reserved judgement. Only a few (such as Merkel and Krause) agreed with Johnston and were vindicated as new techniques confirmed Johnston's theory. In doing so, Johnston quietly ushered in a new evolutionary perspective into neuroanatomy.

However, the question of the origin of the cells remains. Are these seemingly displaced cells some form of primary sensory neurons reabsorbed from a ganglion into the brain, or could they perhaps be a remnant of an evolutionarily simpler sensory system – an atavism – somehow trapped within the brains of land-dwelling reptiles, birds and mammals?

Personally, I like the idea that this is a remnant of an earlier kind of nervous system trapped in the brain of a sophisticated vertebrate. I can imagine a scenario where the young larvae of a new kind of fish, armed with the ability to chew its food, adapted the sensory cells of its more ancient forebears to sense the pressure of its bite. As the rest of the body discarded this ancestral sensory system, first during the metamorphosis into adulthood, then altogether as vertebrates colonised land, the primitive sensory cells attached to our teeth somehow got left behind – too useful to replace, fit for purpose, with no need to upgrade. Their role in allowing the animal to feed was perhaps simply too essential or complicated to replace in mid-life. Whatever the reason, this piece of history became embedded in all our brains.

Atavism (the retention of hidden ancestral traits) may also have entered the thoughts of another neuroanatomist working on the sensory systems of juvenile lampreys and fish some years before Johnston. He published his observations in 1878, almost twenty years before Johnston's survey of mesencephalic neurons across multiple fish species. The cells that this young neuroanatomist, Sigmund Freud (1856–1939), called *hinterzellen* were a unique population of primitive sensory neurons that somehow survived into adulthood in the lamprey. And when Freud turned his attention to the nervous system of the freshwater crayfish, an invertebrate, he found neurons that were remarkably similar to the *hinterzellen* he had just described in animals with a backbone. Did Freud stop and wonder whether his *hinterzellen* were evolutionary throwbacks – atavisms?

The retention of ancestral traits, hidden instincts and atavisms were a hallmark of Freud's later psychoanalytical theories. The origins of these dark ideas of lurking primitive desires and behaviours were unclear and he was often criticised for not having provided evidence to support his theories. But perhaps the atavisms that he went on to explore in our sub-conscious mind were a reflection of earlier evidence he first considered as a neuroanatomist.[vii]

We will never know whether Freud privately recognised or speculated about brain cells. For reasons that are not entirely clear, he destroyed all his notes and diaries when he left neuro-anatomy behind and moved on to study the human mind. But I wonder whether the similarity between the nerve cells that he drew in the lamprey and then in the crayfish, and the possibility of anatomical atavism, were buried deep in Freud's subconscious only to emerge later in his famous theories of the mind – a throwback to his younger self.

Cell 5

The leech neuron and the nerve net

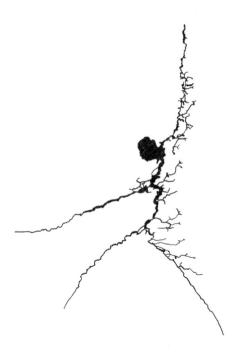

One of the three types of sensory cell in the nerve cord of a medicinal leech. This T-cell responds to a light touch on the surface of the leech's skin. Parts of the cell stretch out to link the knots of cells that control each body segment. To some early anatomists this apparent continuity across segments made leech neurons a seemingly vast continuum of fused cells.

More than 500 million years ago, the last common ancestor of vertebrates and invertebrates swam in oceans. Animals with and without backbones lived side by side and at different times; both made their own independent exploration of land. The invertebrates made it onto land first and one branch evolved into the multitude of flying and flightless insects that colonised every conceivable niche. Vertebrates followed many millions of years later, swapping fins for limbs, gills for lungs, exploiting their internal skeleton to become giants in comparison with their insect cousins. Both took the basic rudiments of a nervous system that had become such a successful innovation in water. They followed their own paths, finding similar solutions but building arrays of brain cells mediating sensation and driving behaviour.

When you draw the brain cells of invertebrates you can feel the evolutionary distance between them and us. Our brains are undoubtedly related but something about the way that cell branches divide, the angles and the lengths between nodes, the way the finest arms stretch to touch their neighbours betrays their alienness. The fundamental principles of axons and dendrites are confused, less easy to read. Is this even the right way to describe their form or are we imposing a vertebrate view of the world on a system of neural connectivity that has grown independently sophisticated?

My own drawings of invertebrate brain cells took me back to a technique that pre-dated the photography on which I later relied. It was in the first days of my becoming a neuroscientist and I was trying to find a way to perfect the method of doing the seemingly impossible – injecting a single, microscopic brain cell with a dye that will fill its most fragile thread-like extensions. The neurons in a leech were huge compared with the retinal ganglion cells that I was hoping to stab with my glass micropipette: beach balls rather than tennis balls. They were sturdy enough to survive being filled, not with fluorescent Lucifer yellow, but a solution of large protein – an enzyme derived from the horseradish that would turn black as ink when exposed to a toxic mix of hydrogen peroxide and carcinogenic diamino benzidine.

Once converted into a pigment, the dye within the brain cell can sit for years on a shelf (much like the famous Golgi stain), whereas the more ephemeral fluorescence eventually fades. It also allows the use of a device called the camera lucida to trace the shape of the neuron directly from the slide without the need for photography. The camera lucida, or drawing tube, superimposes the image of the paper that you are drawing on over the view down the microscope. You can literally trace directly what you see.

The act of drawing in this way is a complex three-dimensional dance under the microscope. It is magical – a little like the Pepper's Ghost illusion in the Victorian fairground or like illusory performers from the past conjured onto the stage in modern concerts, where a three-dimensional projected image forms seemingly miraculously in space through the precise interplay of light and glass.

The fingers of one hand are gripped on the microscope focus knob; the other holds a black ink-filled pen poised over the paper under the drawing tube, sticking out at right angles from the microscope. As I look through the eyepieces I can see both what is under the microscope – a beautiful and delicate leech neuron – and the bright, white paper under the heel of my hand. The choreography of balancing light, focus and mark-making begins. If there is too much light on the paper coming through the drawing tube, it glares through the eyepieces and the image of the cell is obscured. If there is too much light passing through the glass slide, then I cannot see the lines that I have drawn. When the balance is right, my hand is ghostly and the ink is filling in shadows. I turn the focus to bring a frond of black into sharp relief and fill the shadow with ink and continue, moving up and down, tracing lines through microscopic space. Eventually I take my eyes from the eyepieces and the delicate fronds of a leech neuron merge to form a complete cell on the page.

The camera lucida achieves the same aim as the camera obscura, invented in the sixteenth century, which enabled artists to create paintings and drawings with accurate proportions. In a darkened room or light-proof box, a single, pinprick-sized hole projects a startlingly bright and colourful, inverted image onto the facing surface: the three-dimensional drama of the outside world turns into a two-dimensional moving picture. It seems likely that this systems of lenses and mirrors allowed Jan Vermeer, an art dealer and painter from Delft, to produce his prized and stunningly precise paintings of Dutch everyday domesticity. The popularity of the camera obscura as a tool for the amateur Victorian painter was wide-spread and became the foundation for photography. Something about this older delight of viewing the world as captured and reduced into a two-dimensional frame lies at the heart of film and photography.

The camera lucida was patented in 1806 by William Hyde Wollaston (1766–1828), one of a band of astoundingly prolific tinkerer scientists who drove the evolution of the Royal Society through forays into medicine, metallurgy, physics, chemistry and industry. Wollaston was a member of the Board of Longitude, who administered (but never awarded) the prize for the accurate calculation of position at sea – a challenge met by John Harrison's famous chronometers. Wollaston's experiments with electricity and the invention of a well-guarded technique for purifying platinum had made him famous and wealthy, but the camera lucida was a hobby, a passion with not much commercial promise that had been made possible by experiments in prisms. Wollaston found that by gluing two wedges of the crystalline calcite glass together, he could collect images from two different sources and superimpose them in the same visual plane. For the microscope, the Wollaston prism would allow the hand, pen and the neuron to be superimposed.

Wollaston's prisms are still exploited in a variety of different guises. The science of interferometry relies on optically superimposing images to discover infinitesimal flaws.[i] However, the camera lucida itself seems as old-fashioned as a magic lantern and these once common drawing tubes are now largely relegated to the laboratory cupboard. Just as the camera obscura evolved into photography, the ability to capture images through a microscope onto a camera or a computer means that the understanding of form by directly drawing at the microscope has disappeared. But something is lost because we no longer draw what we see down the microscope. This is hard to define but there is a sense that the understanding that comes through the movement of arm, hand and eye is closer to knowing a form than being able to measure it.

As I follow the thready tendrils of the leech sensory cell with my pen, I can feel the difference between the delicate tracery of its fronds and the stout branches of a vertebrate Purkinje cell. They are draped across each other like the rope threads of a mop. If thought has a shape, then the shape of thinking in a leech is different to that in fish, reptiles, birds and mammals. Feeling this difference in the sensual act of drawing is not the same as knowing that this really is the case, though it seems incredibly important as I sit at the microscope.

But in some ways the answer is simple. The neuron is a physical manifestation of the flow of information. Perhaps it is surprising that there is any similarity at all between the neurons encased within the leech, a limbless segmented worm, and those within a warm-blooded vertebrate that shapes can build and communicate. If an alien species washed up on our planet, would it have brain cells? Would they look the same as ours? Does thought have to be shaped this way?

The leech nervous system does not have a central brain but repeats as a series of similar segments along its body length. The segments are added one at a time in the embryo, each with the same basic set of neurons. My neuron was one of the medium threshold sensory neurons – a light touch on the skin is just enough to cause it to become excited. Between the ganglia, the sensory neurons send longer connections. However, the distinction between axon and dendrite is unclear and it disappears as the dye I injected becomes fainter. I feel it's a single cell. The thread-like processes within the ganglion that contains all the nerve cell bodies have blind endings, but what happens in the next segment? Where does this cell end? As I trace the thin filament that stretches to the next cluster of cell bodies in the next leech segment, I'm not so sure.

I have come across this before – the boundary between being able to see the edges of what I am drawing and what begins to seem improbable. An anxiety creeps in. This does not feel right. I must have missed a gap. I go back and check. The cell cannot be continuous with its neighbour; there must be a break in the line. I know it will have a definitive stop. The cell will end, and I accept this because of a theory proposed by Theodor Schwann in the 1820s who proposed that living creatures are composed of aggregates of cells.

Schwann's cell theory applies to nearly all things living and certainly to all animals. Fungus and mushrooms are outliers in the plant world with their continuous tubes of cellular stuff with multiple cell nuclei. But these fungal tubes without boundaries (syncytial) are confined to the remote branches of a non-animal world.

In the minds of most scientists in the middle of the nineteenth century, there was one part of the animal that seemed fungal and syncytial. The nervous system, with its dense meshwork of fibres and impenetrable soup of cell nuclei seemed very un-cell-like when viewed through the latest microscopes. Although Schwann's theory held true for skin, liver, kidneys and muscle, the brain seemed to be an exception – a mass of ordered and seamless fibres that matched the coherent and unitary nature of our thoughts and consciousness.

The intellectual appeal of the brain as a single structure found resonance with a philosophy of mind that emerged with the eighteenth-century German Enlightenment philosopher Immanuel Kant (1724–1804). The precise nature of thought was a question for philosophy rather than science. The detailed anatomical structures of the brain and spinal cord were of less interest than the collective output of whatever was in this black box. However, this was about to change with the emergence of the field of neuroscience. The debate that forged neuroscience would be about the existence of cells in the brain. Was the mechanism of thought based in a continuum or was it fractured into millions of individual components, perhaps each capturing and processing a part of our thinking – our brains as a community rather than an individual?

What part does the leech have to play in this debate? Medicinal leeches are distinctive: a pattern of orange on green pigmentation, which reminds me of a New Mexico rug in its geometric angled pixels, with powerful swimming muscles and a sinister round, toothed and saw-like mouth. My medicinal leeches came from tanks in South Wales where enterprising Roy Sawyer, the leech man with connections across the globe, had established a flourishing business. Unfed, medicinal leeches shrink to earthworm proportions but after a meal they became large, intimidating and fast swimming creatures. But it wasn't until I spent a summer in Borneo, partly spurred on by my drawing in the laboratory, that I understood why leeches were sought-after laboratory partners. In the forests of Southeast Asia, the leeches live on land rather than in water; they perch, small and emaciated, patiently waiting for a rare chance to feed. As you pass by, the creatures follow your movement – is it the heat, the smell? – and somehow, despite all the care to seal holes and gaps in clothing, wearing the leech socks that tie tightly below the knee, they find a way to your skin. Like their larger, aquatic medicinal cousins, the little terrestrial leech can attach itself without the knowledge of the unwary scientist. Its secret power is in its saliva that contains the most effective natural anticoagulant known: hirudin. While the leech sits undetected, hirudin keeps the blood from clotting and the leech drinking.

Roy's tanks bred leeches for this property of anticoagulation and the promise of restoring blood flow to severed digits by drawing circulation back into potentially dying tissue using carefully placed leeches. These same properties made leeches indispensable for all the wrong reasons – for over hundreds of years deployed in the mistaken and potentially disastrous practice of drawing blood to treat a range of illnesses.

Effective blood-letting required clotting to be blocked. The European leech, *Hirudo medicalis*, which was less voracious and less painful than New World leeches, had been plundered from freshwater ponds in central Europe to the extent that it had become an endangered species by the time its use peaked in the 1830s. A roaring international trade in leeches resulted in them being harvested, exported or smuggled as contraband. More than 6 million were ordered for hospitals in Paris alone.

When scientists started looking for species to investigate neural anatomy, they turned to a creature that was already commonplace in institutions across the globe and found a segmented nerve cord packed with nerve fibres to investigate. Perhaps the most skilled of these was a Hungarian anatomist, István Apáthy (1863–1922), who travelled to Naples and the Stazione Zoologica marine biology research institute, to apply his skill at tissue staining to the leech.

Apáthy arrived as an explosion of new dyes and processes

offered a trove of different ways to pickle and stain the leech nervous system: precious metals, new organic pigments and poisons; gold chloride, methylene blue, osmium and mercury. As Apáthy tried and tested these new approaches he became increasingly convinced that the leech nerve cord was a network of unbroken and continuous threads. His insights chimed with what the German physician Joseph von Gerlach (1820–1896), who finessed his staining with gold, was finding. To Apáthy's eyes, the finest tendrils of each fibre were clearly fused into a dense network which he dubbed a 'protoplasmic continuum'. Camillo Golgi, who saw blind-ending dendrites as tubes for feeding the continuum joined with Apáthy in a scientific consensus that the fibres (which would become known as axons) stretching across the nervous system formed a single continuous net that linked all of the brain in a 'reticulum'.

One of the reasons that Apáthy was convinced of the existence of the reticulum is that he could see inside the leech neuron to the protein skeleton that supported its form. Working with every technical advance and studying cells whose bodies were twenty or thirty times larger than those in a human brain, Apáthy was able to see into the structure of the cell itself. Apáthy's cell skeleton neurofibrils became his focus of intense study and with that focus came a belief that his neurofibrils extended, unbroken, through and beyond cell boundaries as a continuum, similar to a miniature electrical cord. Sensation at the skin of the leech was relayed through to muscular contraction in the body wall by an unbroken fusion of microscopic fibres.

Apáthy was obsessive and a perfectionist. It took a further eight years after leaving Naples to complete his experiments, collate his observations and summarise his thoughts before his

200-page article on the finer structures of the nervous system was published. However, by the time his magnum opus was delivered, the scientific world had moved on. The beautiful and detailed conception of the reticulum would run up against something new and contradictory – a burgeoning theory of the neuron doctrine: a brain composed of individual cells, each holding its own fragment of thought.

As Apáthy worked tirelessly on the production of his great work, three key figures emerged as champions of a cell theory for the brain: Auguste Forel, Wilhelm His and Fridtjof Nansen, whom Apáthy had encountered as a young doctoral student in Naples many years before. Each approached the challenge of a cell theory from a different perspective and a different set of passions that I like to imagine shaped their thinking.

Forel (1848–1931), a psychiatrist and anatomist, based his attack on the reticular theory on his observation that when a nerve was damaged, the fibres within it died. However, the spread of the degeneration stopped abruptly at the first cell bodies. If the brain was a continuous net, he reasoned that there should be no breaks in the transmission of degeneration. If the brain was made up of cells, however, there must be gaps across which the degeneration would not pass. Cells were in close contact, no doubt, but not fused. A simple contact was enough to transmit information between nerve cells. There was no continuous mesh but rather a vast population of individuals communicating with each other to create a collective mind.

This view might have been almost subconsciously re-inforced through Forel's passion for ants whose colonies display what is as close as possible to a collective intelligence. As a high school student, Forel had failed his first attempt to gain entry to the medical school in Lausanne. Searching for something to occupy an empty summer, he set about collecting and cataloguing different species of ant from across Switzerland. Later, after twenty years serving as the director of an asylum at Burghölzli, Forel returned to his earlier passion and completed a monumental five-volume work on the social structure and behaviour of colonies, *The Social World of Ants*, speculating on how their world mimicked human society.

Forel was well aware how his observations of cellular degeneration challenged the dominant theories of reticularists. And so he was frustrated when Wilhelm His published similar conclusions about the cellular nature of the brain just a year before in 1886. In contrast to Forel's background in psychiatry, His was an embryologist and came at the problem from looking at the development of brain cells.[ii] He saw that the young brain was composed of individual ovoids, much like germinating seeds. As the embryo grew, forming a distinct head and extending paddle-like limbs that become tipped with fingers, so nerve cells extended finger-like processes to penetrate these structures. If each brain cell started as a single ovoid then the mesh of fine processes that made up the adult nervous system must have its origin in individuals. The fused reticulum was an illusion born of complexity. At a simpler, embryonic stage, it was clear that the brain was composed of individual cells.

And then there was Fridtjof Nansen (1861–1930), the third important critic of the reticulum theory and often cited in contemporary accounts as the chief advocate for a theory that the brain was composed of cells rather than a diffuse network. His fleeting, if intense, career in neuroscience is perhaps the most intriguing of three champions of brain cell theory and

Nansen was the only one who likely crossed paths with Istvan Apáthy. By the time of the showdown between the reticularists and proponents of a neuron doctrine at the 1906 Nobel Prize ceremony in Stockholm, Fridtjof Nansen had already moved on from science, finding international recognition as a polar explorer.

Fifteen years earlier, as a new doctoral student in Bergen, Nansen had fallen, it seems almost by chance, into the post of curator of a nearby private natural history museum. Here, he became engrossed in the study of marine parasitic worms (myzostomes). These animals, who attach to and feed off the body fluid of fish, have a reduced – almost residual – nervous system. As he examined the nervous system of myzostomes, Nansen began to doubt the validity of the nerve net theory. Using the best microscope he could afford, with new objective lenses with a resolving power so great and a working distance so small that they nearly touched the glass of the slide, he used a camera lucida to trace nerve cells directly onto stone to make lithographs. What he saw and etched were the visible gaps between the nerve cells.

Fascinated by the nature of the connection between neurons and the apparent lack of a reticulum he started to work his way through different marine creatures: from the sea squirt to the hagfish which, like the lamprey, lay at the boundary of vertebrate and invertebrate animals.[19] At some point, he heard about the new staining technique invented by Camillo Golgi in Northern Italy and resolved to visit him in the summer of 1886 to learn what he could about this breakthrough. On his way back from Pavia, armed with the recipe for the black reaction and convinced that the brain was made of cells, he made a detour to spend the summer at the Stazione Zoologica in Naples.

I like to think this is where the young Norwegian adventurer and soon-to-be polar pioneering explorer found himself: in the company of the reserved and meticulous István Apáthy, who arrived in Naples in the same year. Both were in their twenties and intent on studying the microscopic structure of the nervous system of invertebrates. How could they have avoided each other?

Nansen was already convinced, correctly, that nerve cells were autonomous units, communicating across vanishingly small gaps. Apáthy was wedded to established dogma and everything he saw with his exquisite stains seemed, incorrectly, to prove Nansen wrong. He would spend the next twelve years refining and collecting data to try to disprove Nansen's ideas and put forward his own theory that neurofibril cables ran through the cells connecting the nervous system like a series of taut electrical cords.

Nansen's summer was soon over and he was in a hurry to complete his doctoral studies and move on. Armed with Golgi's stain, he headed back to Bergen and the following summer submitted his thesis. Barely pausing to hear whether he had passed or failed, he rushed almost directly from the examination room to catch a steamer to Greenland where he would make that first successful crossing of the ice cap on skis with hand-drawn sledges. Eight years later he made an unsuccessful attempt on the North Pole. Trapped on the ice for eight months, in a hut he built with his companion Hjalmar Johansen only fifty miles from rescue, I wonder how many times Nansen's mind turned to memories of that warm Italian summer in Naples.

Apáthy stayed on for another four years at the marine biological research station in Naples, reading no doubt of the heroic achievements of the Norwegian summer student who wanted to trash the predominant reticular theory of the day. He returned to Hungary and an illustrious career, but became increasingly interested, like Forel in Switzerland, in applying biology to the solution of human problems.[iii] Unfortunately, like many of their generation, both became champions of the disastrous pseudo-science of eugenics as a means of improving a nation's health. By contrast, Fridtjof Nansen went on to receive the Nobel Peace Prize for humanitarian work after the First World War, introducing the 'Nansen passport' for the stateless and dispossessed refugees. The contrast between the two men seems stark. Nansen on the side of the poor and downtrodden and on the 'right' side of science. Apáthy seduced by eugenics and ending up on the 'wrong' side with Golgi, himself in the thrawl of Cesare Lombroso, the proponent of a discredited theory that criminality was inherited.

Did Nansen and Apáthy find each other's personalities unbearable that summer in Naples? Science is an intensely human pursuit driven by ambitions, passions and prejudices. Nansen's thoughts were half on polar exploration and adventure. Apáthy appeared slower, more diligent and more conservative. When Apáthy finally published his studies in 1897, the exasperation at their incorrect conclusions was barely concealed in a contemporary account: 'A more unsatisfactory condition of knowledge or a more prohibitive hypothesis can scarcely be conceived.'[20] Apáthy's drawings were beautiful but fatally flawed. He had stubbornly failed to acknowledge anyone else's work – and particularly Nansen's.[iv]

Or is it too easy to cast heroes and villains in science for the sake of a story? Here is the vision that I prefer. Two young scientists thrown together in Naples over one warm summer with different backgrounds and hopes but a shared passion for the brain. Apáthy and Nansen sit, with a bottle of wine, legs dangling over the edge of the dock above a blue sea looking over the Bay of Naples on a summer's evening chatting about the ocean, exploration, and what they had seen that day through the microscope, setting the course for their legacy.

Usually, it is history that gradually sidelines scientists to their different camps. Those who fall the wrong side of an argument might find their names becoming more anonymous over time – forgotten by succeeding generations, infrequently referred to, only appearing in historical appraisals such as this one. However, in the story of the brain cell, protagonists were instantly cast as heroes and villains by their contemporaries. The feelings evoked were powerful.

Wind forward to 1906 and Santiago Ramón y Cajal is sitting, fuming inwardly, aghast as he hears Camillo Golgi speak flawed science to a captive audience, attacking Cajal's ideas after a Nobel Prize ceremony that defined their respective histories. He feels that Golgi has ignored, like Apáthy, all the evidence around him and, perhaps more importantly, the evidence of his own eyes.

At around the same time, Sigmund Freud is destroying the notebooks from his neuroanatomy career. One theory is that they detailed his own adherence to the nerve net theory a full ten years before Nansen and Apáthy converged on Naples. Had Freud's theories of the brain's organisation, which shaped the development of his psychoanalysis, sprung from a misconception? Was there a fallacy so substantial, so grievous that had to be erased from his own records or risk being on the wrong side of history?[v]

There seems to be something exceptional about the

93

intensity of this debate. It is not the normal weighing up of evidence over time, a difference of opinion that arises because techniques are flawed or results are contaminated. It is not even because of a bias in the interpretation of data. The origins of the passions around the reticulum come from the belief in what each scientist saw. This was not a debate about understanding – it was a challenge to what each knew to be true.

As I draw my invertebrate leech neuron, as Apáthy and maybe Nansen and Freud had done before, there is no room for doubt that the processes sticking out at different angles have a defined end. If I can't quite see the join (it appears a little ambiguous), my pen will break the connection between the filaments. That's the inbuilt logic of knowing this is a brain cell. This is what I see.

Questioning visual judgement is a skill rarely taught in science and the origins of that judgement are rarely examined. When I look down a microscope, it is easy to understand why I see brain cells and not a reticulum. Brain cells are what I know to be there. My eyes would refuse to see anything different.

But in the 1890s there were no precedents to shape such subconscious judgement, only the individual experiences of its protagonists. The explanation often given is that reticularists were influenced by concepts of mind that rested on networks of activity. Neuron doctrine followers saw the intellectual roadblock that this erected, given the increasing and compelling evidence for the localisation of function in different areas of the brain. They also had Schwann's cell theory as a powerful influence.

However, I wonder how much of these decisions so critical in the moment were shaped long before. Apáthy's innate conservatism did not allow him to think beyond what the leading reticularists of the day thought and the 'presumed necessity of continuous structure'.[21] Forel, on the other hand, saw in the colonies of the ants that he studied how individuals could come together to make a collective will. Nansen was open to exploration and novelty.

One episode from Cajal's autobiography that always sticks with me is how, as a rebellious twelve-year-old, he constructed a den on a neighbour's rooftop where he could escape to read fiction and draw freely – activities that were disapproved of by his austere father. From there, he spotted a library in a room above the next-door bakery. Creeping in while the pastry chef and family were asleep, Cajal borrowed, one book at a time, *The Hunchback of Notre Dame*, *The Three Musketeers*, *Robinson Crusoe* and other contraband stories. The story of Crusoe, stranded on what appeared to be a deserted island – virgin territory – particularly struck Cajal as significant in his later autobiography: 'to gaze upon scenes untouched by the hand of man, adorned with their original flora and fauna'.[22] Did Cajal find in the landscape of the brain the same untouched landscapes that Nansen risked his life to find in the far North? Could this thirst for seeing something new, previously unseen, have primed the judgement to be more rebellious?

Much later in life, Cajal wrote a self-help book for young investigators that was a guide to both the laboratory and to life. Happily married himself, he devoted some paragraphs to the correct choice of wife. The presumed virtues and betrayed prejudices tell us as much about nineteenth-century Spanish culture as science. However, there is an unusual and strikingly modern reflection on objectivity later echoed by the twentieth-century photographer Richard Avedon (1923–2004). Like Cajal, Avedon documented the diverse characters and his most well known are the extraordinary, gritty portraits collected from across the American West that inspired his most famous quote: 'Sometimes I think all my pictures are just pictures of me. My concern is . . . the human predicament; only what I consider the human predicament may simply be my own.'[23] Cajal's reflection on the impossibility of objectivity reads more like an artist than a scientist: 'All description, no matter how objective and simple it may seem, constitutes personal interpretation – the point of view of the author himself.'[24]

Cell 6

A universal brain cell

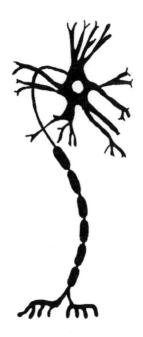

The idealised form of the archetypal neuron depicted by Lewellys Barker. Copied thousands of times, most pictures based on his diagram share the features of stubby dendrites, a curving axon and sausage-like swellings representing the truncated myelin-rich arms of specialised glial cells. This drawing is fairly close to the 1897 version in Barker's book, but a vast range of increasingly abstracted versions appear in popular visual culture and in school textbooks.

When I was at school I wasn't really interested in science. I liked drawing but I wasn't strong enough or insightful enough to pursue art. I enjoyed understanding how things worked and building models. Biology was as close as I could get to using drawing in everyday lessons. Many lessons involved drawing from life: a flower structure, a dissected rat, the view of a thin wafer of onion skin under the microscope. Many more involved reconstructing diagrams from textbooks. Perhaps if I had seen a real brain cell I would instantly have been grabbed by neuroscience but the first brain cells we draw, that we all draw at school, were confusing, isolated creatures, looking a little like a stranded piece of seaweed, a million miles from the elaborate and intricate forms that in reality crowd the brain.

More than that, we only ever drew one brain cell. It is a brain cell that is instantly recognisable from textbook pages to school lesson plans to a host of popular cultural representations of the neuron. And it is a brain cell that does not exist in real life.

Stubby dendrites widen dramatically as they merge with a fried egg. Hanging off the fried egg and trailing to the right, a bunch of sausages appear to be dragged along the ground and at the end is a hand with multiple stubby thumbs. This is the brain cell and its component parts, often not assembled in the right order when reproduced by students in the essays that I mark, sometimes a jumble of bits and often with a strange snowflake regularity that just isn't organic.

I have to admit that, like the students I encounter at the university where I teach neuroscience, none of this made any sense before I had seen my first brain cell down the microscope. The dendrites taper delicately to fine points that seem to be reaching for something close by, maybe just beyond their grasp. The axons are a stouter cable, built with more purposeful rigidity to carry a message faithfully onwards. The cell body holds it all together, tensed against some invisible pull. The elegant unity of form and function had somehow been lost or could not be conveyed in the drawing of a neuron that I and thousands of others had learned. We spill out the drawing, learned by rote, but completely miss the concept and the beauty.

When I first came across this phenomenon, my immediate thought was that, once exposed to seeing a brain cell using a microscope to peer deep into the tissue, students would start to change the way they drew. It was long after my first encounters with neurons that it occurred to me that my neuroscientist colleagues were all drawing different brain cells when they sketched out a problem or an idea. They each tended to have a favourite, almost always different to the fried egg and sausages drawn by school and new university students, and that favourite was almost a signature. I teamed up with colleagues and we began a systematic survey, trying to find whether it was some sort of magical exposure to research perspective that shaped these signatures. Would students change the way they drew their brain cells – abandon the textbook image that we all learned – if they tasted a small fragment of that culture of research?[i]

A small group of us became gripped with this exploration of the visual constraints that shaped our cell signatures and we were soon asking everyone to draw brain cells on paper, on pebbles collected at the beach, from the most senior scientists to the class of eleven-year-olds. At some point it became clear that for the scientists at least, the drawing of a brain cell was not so much a reflection of research experience but of a research question. What is it in the brain cell that you might want to discover? And how do you explain that need to others?

Without a question to ask, the neuron drawing can happily rest in its state of fried eggs and sausages. It is an instantly recognisable form whose finer details do not matter, only the whole. We can jumble the details a little, make the sausages a little fatter or thinner, the stubby fingers a little longer, the yolk a little smaller, but its symbolic meaning remains. Where did this resilient archetypal brain cell – the universal brain cell that is repeated over and over from textbook to student essay to children's book to public health leaflet – come from?

Back in 1891, at the cusp of the brain cell era, an ambitious Canadian doctor, Lewellys Barker (1867–1943), arrived in Baltimore. He had just graduated from the University of Toronto and was keenly aware that in moving south to Maryland he could put himself at the heart of a movement in medicine that would radically change the way in which doctors would be trained across the world.

Barker had been recruited to a new kind of training programme (a 'residency') by William Osler, one of the founding professors of the new medical school called Johns Hopkins. In this revolutionary system the 'resident' would, for the first time, receive specialist training within the hospital under the supervision of more senior doctors. Barker excelled in this innovative environment, rising rapidly through the academic ranks to become Professor of Anatomy in Chicago at the age of thirty-three. When Osler crossed the Atlantic to direct medical studies at the University of Oxford in 1905, it was the tall, handsome and effortlessly gracious Barker, now in his late thirties, who returned to Baltimore to take his place.

It was not the clinical training of the residency that had allowed Barker to thrive. In fact, he was not much of a practising clinical doctor at all, a fact that subsequently made his appointment to Osler's post controversial. When Barker first arrived in Baltimore, the new medical school at Johns Hopkins was trialling the idea that medicine and research could be combined into a single career within a medical school. Doctors could be recruited to the faculty where they would become, for the first time, full-time academics with both teaching obligations and research interests. And it was in this role that Barker had been appointed an associate professor, abandoning the private practice that would conventionally have paid his salary. Embracing this climate of research, and mentored by Franklin Mall, a passionate advocate of scientific approach to medicine, Barker threw himself into studying the nervous system.

Brain cells and the brain were the things to be looking at if you were young and curious in the 1890s. Barker worked alongside a new intake of pioneering female medical undergraduates including Florence Sabin, who later became the first female professor of anatomy and the first female department head at New York's Rockefeller University, and Gertrude Stein, who would leave medicine behind to find fame as a leading figure of a Parisian avant-garde of art, jazz and literature.

Barker's first decade in Baltimore was a period of intense industry. Although his experiments made little impact, he could see that a surge in discovery spurred on by Golgi and Cajal in Europe needed to be brought together in a new venture: the first neuroscience textbook. Working at enormous pace and gathering as much as he could from the publications that began to spill from the international laboratories, he assembled a giant compendium of brain anatomy and neuroscience ideas that was published in 1897, only six years after he arrived at Johns Hopkins.

This monumental work is now long out of print and largely forgotten. Barker's encyclopaedic book, *The Nervous System*, does not sit on open library shelves and it is unlikely to have been studied for many years. However, buried within its pages is a decisive contribution to how we have all viewed the brain since: the first, definitive diagram of a brain cell with its stubby, truncated dendrites, curving axon and a cell body like a fried egg.

The illustration that forms Figure 17 of his book is an idealised neuron that in its compelling simplicity has long eclipsed Barker's name. The pages of his book are richly illustrated with beautiful examples of cells from different areas of the brain, as well as photographs and sketches directly from the microscope. Together, the strikingly visual work builds a snapshot of the landscape of brain cell discovery in the late 1890s: the material that different scientists were working with and, in showing elaborate brain cell forms, a contentious recognition of their status as individual and indivisible units.

Barker's book is the visual story of development of a brain cell doctrine written, not by a pioneer in the laboratory, but by a contemporary populariser of science.

Figure 17 was a visual representation of a term that itself was an act of cultural appropriation: the neuron. The word was not new: it had been passed around in various forms and applied to different parts of the brain. However, it was a professor in Berlin, Wilhelm von Waldeyer-Hartz, who enshrined it within the phrase 'neuron doctrine' in 1891. Waldeyer's claim to the right to name the brain cell came not from any personal observation or experiment – it was an intellectual property grab. This was no doubt facilitated by his considerable status as full Professor of Anatomy in the science powerhouse of Berlin, but also an uncanny ability to name a concept: just three years earlier he had coined the term 'chromosome'.[ii] Barker wanted to encapsulate Waldeyer's neuron theory visually with a single image that expressed the brain cell as a theory. The picture with its stubby dendrites, its axon with characteristic, irresistible curve and sausage-like wrappings of myelin, has been copied and re-copied many millions of times.

Writing many years later, Cajal bemoaned the fact that Waldeyer had laid claim to a neuron doctrine that had clearly been established by the small band of scientists who had challenged the dominant theory of nerve nets to define a brain cell. But more than Waldeyer's presumption, Cajal would have been unaware that Barker's illustration would rapidly become the symbol of his doctrine. The power of a simple visual icon coupled with the term (the pairing of the simplifying instincts of Barker and Waldeyer) had captured irrevocably the popular conception of a neuron.

What is intriguing is that although Cajal drew many diagrams – explanations of how information might flow through the retina, along the spinal cord between the skin and muscle in a reflex arc – he did not draw *the* diagram, the picture of a single archetypal cell that could encompass his brain cell.

Perhaps this comes back to how what we can see is shaped by what we do. The student makes more or less faithful copies of Barker's neuron in an attempt to make clear their understanding of a concept. The researcher's drawing of a brain cell can be a signature that reflects their research question. Cajal was interested in the details of difference rather than the unifying generality of what a brain cell was. His landscape was a 'magic forest' filled with a myriad of different species and joining together to make a complex functional jigsaw. Perhaps the idea of a single neuron to encapsulate the brain was too foreign to his own vision of the brain to contemplate. After all, which neuron could capture this dazzling diversity? It took a more detached eye, the relative distance of an outsider coming into the field at a critical moment, to say, 'Oh, so this is what you mean . . .'

Barker's lack of attachment to neuroanatomy saw him move rapidly and decisively into a career first as a medical school reformer, a champion of research and interdisciplinary collaboration, and then as a neurologist, finally fulfilling a clinical path that he had temporarily set aside in his twenties.[iii] The legacy of his neuron is somewhat of a paradox. It is a cultural object that transcends the science it sprang from – a shorthand description that is so successful that it almost kills curiosity. Its form has been copied so often that the meaning of its component parts, its authenticity to the real thing so distant and the intellectual excitement from which it sprung have been almost completely obscured.

It is hard to think of the Barker neuron without seeing it as a full stop or a closed door. It is not an object that expresses a question or hypothesis, it has become a symbol for a definition. How many more symbols in science transcend their meaning? Does $e = mc^2$ tell us anything about the speed of light or does its simple elegance stop most of us from asking what it means? A double helix, in all its guises, becomes a token that 'here lie genes' while the meaning in its structure, of its peculiar $C2$ symmetry, is known to only a few. The transition of science discovery into symbol does the exact opposite of science itself. It stops the question. It is the cat that killed the curiosity.

Cell 7

Betz's brain cell and the mapping of the cortex

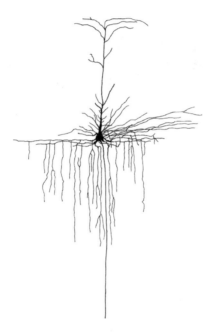

The Betz cell – a pyramidal neuron in layer V of the cerebral cortex. Its massive dendritic tree reaches up to the surface of the brain and stretches sideways to probe and sometimes cling to the trees of neighbouring Betz cells. A wide calibre axon courses down past the deeper structures of the brain (the basal ganglia and thalamus), then through the brainstem to activate the neurons in the spinal cord that control movement.

About a year into studying brain cells as a PhD student, I had a dream about my own brain. In the dream, different regions of my cerebral cortex had gathered together for a party, a weekend away in the countryside. It had the feel of the 1930s about it. Each part of my brain was a two-dimensional jigsaw piece with legs and hands stuck on. It was quite clear that each jigsaw piece had its own character; I'm sure that one piece wore a monocle, plus fours and had a distinguished moustache. There wasn't much plot to the dream, although it was excitingly vivid. The jigsaw pieces were holding conversations: nothing interesting or insightful, it was simply chat. My friend Isobel told me that I had been overdoing my time in the dark of the laboratory.

I had been doing late nights trying to catch up. Neuroscience is a vast subject and my knowledge was patchy, particularly about the cortex. The cerebral cortex is the big highly folded part of the central nervous system we think of when we think of the brain. Its ridges and grooves (gyri and sulci) define our concept of braininess. The bigger, the more folded, surely the better? What made no sense to me was how any single point on this vast landscape of densely packed brain cells could represent a thought or fragment of thought. It did not help that the cortex was made up of layers. This, by contrast, seemed to make the problem worse. Which of these layers was significant? Which brain cell held the thought or action in its grasp? A single point on this folded sheet would represent maybe a thousand cells. Did every cell have an equal opinion? Where were decisions made? It seemed incomprehensible.

A more-or-less universal feature of the cerebral cortex are the six layers of cells, numbered I–VI from top to bottom. In one of these layers, a towering, architecturally elaborate brain cell with a pyramid-shaped cell body shoots upwards into an overarching dendritic tree that spreads upwards and outwards into the overlying four layers of neurons. The pyramidal layer V neuron has a central role in the jigsaw because it gathers the voices of the cells in its immediate orbit. It alone is responsible for communicating with those parts of the central nervous system that directly control how we move, talk and interact with the world. Pushing through the layers of cortical circuitry the layer V pyramidal neuron is the gothic, skyscraping monolith. Its dendrites sample the chatter between layers collecting, integrating and finally launching signals along their monumental axons. This is thought into action, the fingers typing, the lips moving. Signals race downwards, through a funnel of connections that shoot through the brainstem and along the spinal cord.

The smaller inhabitants of the cortex that cluster around the pyramidal neuron include cells whose job is to send signals to other communities around their own layer V neuron – a host of smaller neurons that monitor and refine the streams of information that fly across the surface of the brain. Cells in different strata are sending signals between each other.

Information is exchanged between nearby structures lying just below the cortex. It is a busy hum of information and the layer V cell stretches itself upwards, in contact with all that is going on. Some signals urge the pyramidal neuron to respond, others urge caution and suppress the chatter.

At some point, enough information is gathered by the dendrites of the pyramidal cell that the cell body is forced into action and a volley of impulses is fired. This is the moment that we speak, reach out to touch, display our consciousness to the world.

The fascination of many neuroscientists with the cortical pyramidal neuron is in part its size, partly its connections and partly the cathedral qualities of its form. It is a central organising pillar within the layers of the cortex. Seen through the lens of this towering cell, the cortex is a massive citadel of layer V neurons, attended by the local communities of cells in the other layers. The layer V neuron also has a vital part to play in the story of cortical localisation: how different parts of the cerebral cortex were first identified and then given functional identities.

The six layers of the cortex are found in all mammals and pyramidal cells are a universal feature, varying in relative size both between species and within the cortex. Some types are found only in particular kinds of animals, such as the Meynert cell in the human. It has a single, stately, unbranching dendrite that pushes upwards to end in a firework arc, a spray of tendrils. The base of the main trunk is so densely covered in miniature spines that it appears almost furred.

However, by far the largest of all layer V cells in the human brain sits just in front of the longest groove in the brain. This groove marks a line between the front and back part of the cortex and is known as the central or Rolandic sulcus, the boundary between two of its four lobes, the frontal and parietal. In the ridge, or gyrus, that lies in front of this central sulcus, the cell bodies of the pyramidal neurons dwarf the other layer V cells around them. Not only are they more than ten times larger but whereas in other pyramidal cells, smaller dendrites emerge from the bottom half of the pyramid-shaped cell body, the same dendrites here shoot out in an explosion of branches. Their size allowed them to stand out enough to be recognised by the Ukrainian scientist Vladimir Betz (1834–1894), who found them and after whom they are named.

Betz was a difficult colleague – a trait that may have ultimately hastened his downfall and deprived him of the support he needed when politics interrupted his science. He was highly educated and articulate but displayed his irritability too easily and did not suffer fools gladly.[25] He was an obsessive technical innovator and perfectionist who preferred to install his own printing press at home rather than give the oversight of reproducing the images of his drawings to any publisher. However, his passion and perfectionism in his teaching made him a favourite with his students, as his lectures were a source not only of compendious knowledge but also of wide-ranging social insight. It was significant that he was also an intensely proud Ukrainian. This national pride was ultimately his academic undoing in Kiev.

Betz had risen rapidly within the ranks of academics at St Vladimir's University to extraordinary professor at thirty-four, only to find himself shunned and excluded twenty years later at the celebration of the fiftieth anniversary of founding of the university. His fault had been to court disfavour with officials within the Russian empire by co-authoring a history of the Cossacks that was an overt celebration of Ukrainian culture. It was perhaps the excuse that was needed to get rid of a troublesome figure in the faculty. At the age of fifty-six, he found himself ejected from his position and his laboratory and became physician to the South-Western Russian Railway. Four years later he died of heart disease.

Betz worked with a sticky red dye, ammonium carminate or carmine, that clings to the bodies of cells and is washed out from the gaps between. It was the best cell stain available at the time, years before Golgi's black reaction, but it could never do more than reveal the cell bodies of the densely packed cortex. To do this effectively, the brain had to be sliced into extraordinarily thin wafers. Betz's technical brilliance first involved a chemical process to preserve and stiffen the brain to just the right extent. He then constructed a frictionless knife whose concave surface faced the brain. Its convex upper surface was covered with a thin surface of water, which Betz gently pushed over the knife by blowing through a thin Indian rubber tube held between his lips.

Betz neurons have a peculiar, plant-like form. The burst of horizontal dendrites, like the creeping tendrils of a vine, are sometimes wrapped tightly around the dendrites of smaller neighbours. These tight, intertwined ropes bring the membranes of adjacent cells together, but they do not pass information; it is simply an embrace. Sometimes the horizontal dendrites shoot outwards across the cortical sheet into neighbouring communities of cells, perhaps taking advantage of a gap left by the loss of a neighbouring Betz cell, sometimes downwards into deeper layers like tap roots drawing nutrients from an underground reservoir.

However, none of this elaborate structure was visible to

Vladimir Betz. His discovery, made by soaking the brain in brilliant red carmine, was made twenty years before Camillo Golgi's black reaction revealed the dendritic trees of these towering cells. It seems likely that Betz never saw the intricate detail of their extraordinary giant pyramidal cell architecture. All that he could see was the huge size of their triangular cell body and the intimation of a stout axon, extending downwards from its base.

In contemporary science, technical advances often accompany an almost magical ability to manipulate genes and molecular structure to make a brain glow green, red or blue. Proteins harvested from jellyfish or enzymes recovered from exotic bacteria, isolated, reproduced and inserted into the genes of another animal propel discoveries. For Betz technical innovation consisted of cutting the thinnest and most consistent slices of the brain. Even though I can appreciate this, the image of Betz receiving the Progress Medal at the Vienna World Exposition of 1873 for his superior slicing is still a peculiar thought; it conjures images of the Italian delicatessen next to my children's ballet classes.

Betz's uniform and precise slices allowed him to see not only the 'nests' of his giant cells, each regularly spaced from the next, but also that these giant neurons were only found in one place – the gyrus in front of the central sulcus. Could the single, extruding narrow protrusion out of the bottom of the cell be a wire? Betz became convinced that both the size of the cell and the hint of some kind of output might mean that this was the cell that connected the brain all the way to the spinal cord.

Betz's brilliantly coloured prize-winning specimens from Vienna, all 2,000 samples that he had taken with him, were gifted to his university. They survived the Russian Revolution and two world wars in an unguarded Kiev anatomy department in a metaphor for the persistence and triumph of knowledge and science over conflict that Betz would have readily appreciated.[i] In a chillingly prescient speech to an anatomy audience during the Franco-Prussian war, Betz bemoaned: 'At the time when the people in western Europe who have reached a high level of civic consciousness are physically beating each other, making barbarism worthy of (the) primitive stages (of human development), we . . . [are] . . . gathered here together to start the fight against these social prejudices that from the cradle till the grave clog man's mind.'[26] His battle would be won by 'microscopes, chemical reactants, the devices of physics, and anatomical samples'.

As Betz gave this speech, the war between France and the Prussian Empire of 1870 interrupted the work of two doctors working together in Berlin, Eduard Hitzig (1838–1907) and Gustav Theodor Fritsch (1858–1927), who had been using electricity to stimulate the brains of dogs. Both volunteered for the Prussian army, but not before a seminal account of their work was published and eagerly poured over by Betz.

Hitzig and Fritsch had found that an electrical stimulus to only the front half of the brain stimulated movement. Putting this fact together with the staining that he had seen with carmine, Betz reasoned that it was his giant cells that were responsible for eliciting movement in muscles many hundreds of millimetres away. He was convinced that the one region of the cortex where they resided (the precentral gyrus) was solely responsible for controlling movement. Although traditions of phrenology had long sought to attribute the lumps and bumps on the skull to particular characteristics of personality and mental function, Betz's idea was an important conceptual step: evidence that the brain itself was divided into different areas by function. Betz had correctly identified what would become known as the primary motor cortex.

The idea that function might be matched to regional subdivisions of the cortex inspired the German neurologist Korbinian Brodmann (1868–1918), in the early 1900s, to look in more detail at the cell boundaries in the cortex. In place of Betz's carmine, he used a vivid purple dye, cresyl violet, developed to study brain degeneration by a psychiatrist, Franz Nissl. Brodmann was interested in the sharp boundaries in cell numbers that could sometimes be found within individual layers in the cortex. By tracing these borders, where a layer would suddenly halve in size while another expanded, territories beyond Betz's motor area began to emerge. Brodmann found that in some regions layer IV disappeared to a thin pencil line; in others pyramidal cells in a thick band were themselves dwarfed by Betz's imperious neurons. By 1907, Betz's division of the brain into two parts – a frontal motor area separated from sensory brain by the central groove or sulcus – had become fifty-two areas defined by Brodmann's meticulous cataloguing of layer thickness.

Although there were distinct differences in the fifty-two regions, there was also an overall uniformity in structure. Underpinning the sharp changes in layer thickness, the number of layers was fundamentally unchanged. The cortex could be said to have a modular organisation – a seemingly endless repetition of layer V cells embedded in a swarm of smaller neurons like worker bees surrounding a myriad of queens.

What is the geography of thought? The cortex uncovered

by Betz, Brodmann and others working with similar dyes was essentially a series of repeated microscopic units; within each area, there was nothing to distinguish the cells holding the memory of a grandmother's or a child's face, the pyramidal neurons that flex a finger or a wrist. However, discovering the function of a particular parcel of cortical territory by its connections was undoubtedly an impossible task – the complexity and redundancy of the wiring defying any logical analysis. Working out which area did what required a different approach that did not rely on brain cell shape and microanatomy.

It was an ophthalmologist working in Tokyo, Tatsuji Inouye (1881–1976), who showed, by meticulously cataloguing battlefield injuries in the Russo-Japanese war in 1904–5, that an individual Brodmann area could contain a functional information map.[27] Inouye saw many casualties where a bullet penetrating the head had left a narrow, straight path through the brain. The war between Japan and Russia saw the introduction of a new weapon, the Russian Mosin–Nagant model 91 rifle, which used small high-velocity bullets. Unlike the bullets of modern warfare, these stayed intact as they passed through the human body and brain. The narrow, perfectly straight tunnels allowed Inouye to pinpoint which parts of the brain had been damaged. He found that when the back of the cortex was damaged, patients reported losing specific parts of their vision.

Inouye accurately mapped the paths of bullets in wound after wound and a pattern began to emerge. The most extreme posterior, 'occipital' part of the cortex (the part that is furthest from the eyes) appeared to have a map of the visual world printed on its surface. However, the map was not a

1:1 representation of space. A far larger area of the occipital cortex seemed to be devoted to the fovea (the part with the highest concentration of retinal ganglion cells and the best visual acuity). This was a revelation: neural maps could be distorted according to the importance of the information that the occipital cortex contained.

Half a century later, an American-Canadian neurosurgeon, Wilder Penfield (1891–1976), found the same distortions spread across the pyramidal cell modules of Betz's motor cortex. Like Inouye, Penfield took advantage of the possibilities afforded by his medical practice. He was a neurosurgeon and a pioneer in using brain surgery to isolate the damaged tissue that could be the focal flashpoint for triggering epileptic seizures. In an approach that is still used today, while Penfield operated, he also assessed whether vital functional areas could be spared by his knife. In doing so, he simultaneously created a detailed map of information processing in the brain.

Penfield's revolutionary approach to his surgery had its origins in Golgi's black reaction. As first a science student and then a medical undergraduate at Princeton, Penfield had long harboured an ambition to win a Rhodes Scholarship to England to study at the University of Oxford – an ambition he realised in 1915. Here, he became a lifelong admirer of William Osler, the Johns Hopkins pioneer and now the Regius Professor of Medicine at Oxford. As the First World War broke out, Penfield abandoned his scholarship to become wound dresser for what he thought would be the duration of the conflict. However, when his ship, the SS *Sussex*, was torpedoed in the Channel, Penfield was blown off the deck, landing on wreckage that saved his life but damaged his knee badly enough for him to return to Oxford and find a fortuitous research project in the laboratory of a pioneer of brain research, Charles Scott Sherrington.

It was with Sherrington that Penfield discovered that cutting the axons of neurons had upstream effects on the microscopic structure of the cell body. Eight years later, as a young neurosurgeon in New York, despairing of the high mortality rates of brain surgery and desperate to understand how the brain healed from cuts made by his knife, he remembered his student observations, and perhaps more importantly the advice that Sherrington gave him to try the techniques perfected by Santiago Ramón y Cajal in Madrid.

In 1924, Penfield took himself with his new wife and young family to Spain for five months to learn the black reaction from one of Cajal's former students, Pío del Río-Hortega (1882–1945), who was an expert on glial cells. Using this technique, Penfield delved into the microscopic wreckage caused by surgery and found, alongside the dying neurons, astrocytes that reacted to damage by forming scars, dragging in the partner blood vessels to make a dense mesh. This scarring could also be caused by an accidental brain injury or a tumour and possibly act as a focus for the initiation of an epileptic seizure.

Penfield's mastery of brain cell staining allowed him to start to make precise surgical attacks on epilepsy, taking enormous care that his patients, anaesthetised but conscious, would suffer as little damage to healthy tissues as possible. He knew that any incision had to be extraordinarily gentle to limit glial scarring. But he could also make sure that he restricted his surgery to the scar that was the epileptic source, limiting the damage to the functioning brain. With the cortical surface revealed, Penfield used small electrical currents to stimulate localised areas of the exposed gyri. As he moved his stimulating electrodes from the top of the gyrus, tracing its meandering surface, one part of the body after another twitched.

Just as bullet wounds had mapped the visual cortex, Penfield's expeditions across the surface of the cortex revealed that the primary motor cortex (the precentral gyrus) had a map of the body painted over its surface. The body was hugely distorted. The legs at the peak of the gyrus were thin and emaciated; the face and tongue, the thumb and the hand occupied huge territories and millions more pyramidal cells.

He named the maps he found after the Latin for little man: a 'homunculus' – distorted versions of our own bodies where the most important functions received the most cortical real estate. Penfield demonstrated in his startling and grotesque homunculi how function was the currency of cortical territory: the more important to us, the larger the space on the precentral gyrus given over to its control.

How do we determine importance? When we look at a homunculus it makes sense. The areas requiring finer control – our facial muscles so important in communicating emotion, our fingers through which we handle our tools – have the largest representation.[ii]

As our ability to see patterns of activity in the brain using techniques such as magnetic resonance imaging first complemented and then swamped the data from studies such as Penfield's, something as astonishing as the homunculus emerged from studies of learning and adaptation. Just as significant functions demand more territory within the cortex and more pyramidal cell output, so any change in the status of a muscle or limb could result in its territory being grabbed by its neighbours.[iii]

The digits of the left hand of a violinist do considerably more work than the fingers of the bow hand. Over time and with training, the size of the hand on the homunculus representing the left-hand side of the body (on the right hemisphere of the cortex) grows larger. It begins to take over some of the modules that belonged to another finger, absorbing the circuitry that was previously used to control a different set of muscles. It is not known whether this is because unused connections are gradually activated or because axons or dendrites start growing into neighbouring territory, as sometimes observed in pyramidal neurons. And the opposite is also true. The cortical maps of two fingers that are bound together, in a way that they can no longer move independently, begin to fuse and eventually merge to become a single digit.

And just as there are maps for movement, there are homunculi for sensation, maps for taste, hearing and even memories. From the late 1930s onwards, as Penfield continued his intricate mapping, probing and testing his patients' brains, hunting for sources of epileptic seizures in his patients, he found that stimulation produced not only movements but also illusions of familiarity and of fear. His explorations ranged away from Betz's motor area and into parts of the cortex where different modules clustered around smaller pyramidal neurons.

Stimulation of the temporal lobe of the cortex, closest to the ear, released isolated, vivid flashbacks in his patients that were far more detailed than normal memories. Deeper under the surface, any tissue that he might have to remove from the hippocampus could result in a devastating condition where new memories could not be added to the brain. Stimulating the amygdala, at the tip of the deep, horn-shaped gyrus of the hippocampus, temporarily turned his patients into automata, not conscious of their surroundings or actions and unable to remember anything about the episode. He asked his patients to talk or sing to him while he probed the boundaries of the cortical areas controlling speech, making sure that as much function as possible could be spared. As he worked, meticulously and carefully, Penfield began to paint the functional colours on top of the brain cell boundaries within cortical layers established first by Betz and then comprehensively by Brodmann. Gradually the areas of the cortex in my dream, which had met up for that country weekend, began to make themselves visible.

And just as these cortical features of my overworked imagination had been talking to each other, drinks in hand, Penfield imagined real, neural conversations that must occur between these areas. Putting these together he came up with a now long-forgotten concept he called the centrencephalic system. To Penfield, this was not an anatomical structure but the sum of the ebb and flow of dialogue between ever-changing circuits. The passage of information between circuits, modules and distinct cortical areas (a centrencephalon) was, for Penfield, a conceptual bridge between the functional maps he had found and that illusive, hard to define and yet intimately familiar phenomenon of consciousness.

Cell 8

The reticulothalamic cell and the seat of consciousness

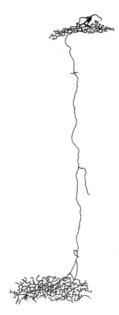

The cell body and dendrites of the reticulothalamic neuron sit at the surface of the thalamus — the nucleus that relays both sensory information and information about cognitive reward and memory to the cortex. The deep axon, tipped with a dense mesh of axon terminals that are inhibitory, gives the potential to shut down information relays with a precision that would inspire a neuronal theory of consciousness.

Consciousness is a notoriously problematic concept for neuroscience. We all know what it is but we consistently fail to give it an adequate definition. It is core to our sense of being, almost self-evidently a property of our brain and yet somehow bigger than the sum of the activity of brain cells. We know what it is to be conscious, but it is impossible to experience someone else's consciousness or determine objectively whether other animals possess what we would understand as the same feeling of being ourselves. We are either conscious beings or we are not. It seems all or nothing; there are no shades of consciousness. But what is its neural signature: where and how do consciousness and the brain cell interact?

For Wilder Penfield, consciousness was an emergent property, something that had no physical home. This is satisfying in that it seems to draw on all our neural faculties to create a unitary beingness, but unbearably vague in that it denies any phenomenon that can be measured or analysed. The opposite approach – finding a material, neural home for consciousness – would seem as fruitless or fantastic as pinpointing the seat of the soul, which René Descartes in the 1600s decided must be the pineal gland, as it was a singular structure in the brain.

As peculiar as it might seem, the hunt for consciousness as something that might be discovered through knowing the personalities and connections of brain cells has nevertheless remained a serious concern for neuroscience.

The groundwork for the search for a neuroanatomical seat of consciousness was laid by Sigmund Freud. Perhaps prompted by the neuroanatomical studies of his youth, he proposed that our brain is able to hold and process thoughts to which we have no direct access, a subconscious mind. Consciousness involves both awareness of an inner self but also the suppression of the activity of at least some part of the brain. It is as much about gathering information as discarding all but the most urgent and relevant.

'Drawing eyes', I have been told, is the way to describe the particular gaze and focus that I have when I have a pen in my hand and am sketching from life. If I'm reminded that I have my 'drawing eyes on', I can stop and recognise that feeling of heightened attention, a cone of concentration. At the heart of putting pen to paper to trace or draw from life is a focus of attention. It's the feeling that has to precede the intricate choreography of muscles that drive the flow of ink. Attending feels different to looking. All senses narrow, not disappearing or shutting off but prioritising a source: the hum of traffic in the background, the square centimetre of paper, the sensation at the fingertips.

The activity of an entire brain is a little like the satellite picture of the earth at night, showing hot spots of artificial lighting in cities and strands of populated connections that link them. The consciousness of our world looks like the night-time activity of millions of homes and businesses. But what is the most significant light in this landscape of illumination – what if it is the single light bulb, a single fragment of a thought? That pool of light, among all the others, is where attention is grabbed for that key fraction of a second. The focus on brain cells allows in the possibility that the seat of consciousness might reside at a cellular scale. It was this question of how to focus on a small cluster of activity and what this might mean for consciousness, that drew an already famous scientist, Francis Crick, to one particular brain cell, the reticulothalamic neuron.

The reticulothalamic neuron has a small bush-like, unspectacular dendritic tree. A thin shell of these brain cells covers the surface of a nucleus of neurons that sits at the heart of the brain – the thalamus. The net (the reticulum) over the thalamus (Latin for inner chamber) is what gives the reticulothalamic neuron its name. Each neuron sends a single axon down into the nucleus below, a little like a fishing line dropping into a deep pond. At the end of the line, axon endings in a focused pool touch a small group of neurons within the body of the thalamus itself. Each cell is a narrow column of information flow from the surface of the nucleus to its core.

It was this architecture that excited Crick. Moreover, reticulothalamic neurons are inhibitory – the kind of brain cell that is able to switch off or slow down the activity in any neuron that its axon touches. The thalamus, Crick knew, was the hub of information flow in the brain and reticulothalamic neurons were a tap potentially controlling this flow.

Francis Crick (1916–2004) was a physicist whose PhD studies on the viscosity of water had been interrupted by the Second World War. After four years of working on the design of magnetic and acoustic mines that could outfox enemy shipping, he abandoned physics and became a born-again biologist. He joined a growing band of exiles from the physical sciences who had become fascinated with the chemical complexity of biological molecules. A key driver was the invention of X-ray crystallography, a technique that used the shadow patterns cast from the scattering of X-ray beams to interpret the shape and symmetry of large and complex molecules. The images that it produced were everywhere in the early 1950s; abstract geometry from the pages of science journals had transferred to wallpaper and fabric designs.[i]

In 1951, Francis Crick met a young American geneticist, James Watson, ten years his junior, and together they resolved to understand the crystal structure of deoxyribonucleic acid (DNA). Understanding the structure of DNA would be central to understanding the genetic code that was somehow bundled up in the tightly coiled DNA molecules that made up chromosomes. The two men struggled to build a model of possible helical structures (that much was known) using small black plates linked with spokes of wire to model chains of amino acids and phosphate molecules, but with no success. However, soon into their partnership they had a huge stroke of fortune when they heard of a single photograph, an X-ray crystallograph taken by Rosalind Franklin (1920–1958) and Maurice Wilkins in London.

Photo 51 is not a spectacular picture when seen alongside the complex and beautiful images of Photos 1–50 and 52 and beyond, each with their filigree patterns of shade and light. But Franklin realised that in the less showy, sparse pattern of islands of shadow of Photo 51 was the unmistakeable signature of a particular kind of symmetry, C2. This could only mean that DNA was made of two spiralling helices. Crick and

Watson were relayed this vital insight, seemingly without the explicit permission of Franklin and Wilkins. It was enough for Crick and Watson to start feverishly completing their model: a spiralling double helix sequence of amino acids, one sequence the complementary image of the other, linked together like a twisting ladder. They published the structure of DNA in a short paper in 1953 and received the Nobel Prize in Physiology or Medicine with Maurice Wilkins in 1962. Rosalind Franklin had died four years earlier at the tragically young age of thirty-eight. Francis Crick, now in his early forties, with the problem of genetic code solved, turned to neuroscience and the brain.

I stumbled across Crick's engagement with consciousness and the neuron in wrestling with how to explain the function of the thalamus (the small cluster of nerve cells at the heart of the brain) to a class of university students. The thalamus is the articulation of the concept of a neural hub. It receives signals from all the senses except for smell, compacts the messages into manageable packets and relays them to the parts of the cortex that deal with hearing, vision, pain, touch. I knew that Crick had become a neuroscientist but not what he had worked on.

Why was the fact that reticulothalamic neurons relayed inhibition so important to Francis Crick? The reticulothalamic neurons, with their dense shrubs of dendrites like the thorny bushes and axons that plunged down into the depths of the thalamus ending in precise dense clusters of tightly packed branches, were perfectly placed to regulate information. It seemed possible that suppressing activity – creating a subconscious brain – might be the route to understanding consciousness. Reticulothalamic neurons, with their distinctive architecture and plugged into the major highway of information in the brain, were ideal candidates for this job.

The concept of inhibition is an important component of the brain cell's world. Inhibition is quick and precise. It can communicate events instantaneously by shutting down a stream of information. It can be the basis of memory but also perception, working alongside neurons that stimulate other cells in a balance that sharpens the patterns of activity across the brain. Neurons that suppress the response or actions of other brain cells are often small and, like reticulothalamic neurons, run local errands. Long axons that end with a role in suppressing activity are relatively rare (Purkinje cells are one example). For the most part, the role of inhibition is local and precise: small, targeted interventions rather than the calming of an entire neighbourhood of cells. In the case of the thalamus, the only source of inhibition is the array of reticulothalamic axons, organised like nuclear fuel rods, plunging deep into the excitable core of the nucleus.

Stopping the flow of information to the cerebral cortex turns out to be a very useful thing to be able to do. It is happening all the time in our brains. Reticulothalamic neurons intervene in the normal flow of sensory information, shutting down the relay at key junctures, to clarify and simplify our world. Five or six times per second, our eyes make rapid, discrete movements – twitches that minutely alter the information entering the retina. This rapid scanning across the visual world not only keeps the disinterested retinal ganglion cells in a state of obedient activity, but also builds up a model of the spaces around us. Every time a twitch (known as a saccade) is made, the thalamus shuts down the flow of signals from the eye to the cortex. The movement of the eye is so fast that these brief shutdowns are needed to shield the brain from what would be a confusing blur of information. When we sleep, the reticulothalamic nucleus comes into play again, suppressing the troublesome noise from our senses.

However, Crick imagined that this would be only part of its job. Having a gatekeeper for sensations from the outside world no doubt affects our conscious experience but does not equate to consciousness. There was another flow of information handled by the thalamus that was of far more interest.

In addition to relaying vision, hearing, touch and pain upwards to the cortex, streams of information arrive at the thalamus from the opposite direction to the flow of sensory information, from the cortex itself. All fifty-two of the cortical areas detailed by Brodmann at the turn of the twentieth century, each with different roles in thinking, planning, emotion, sensing and movement, send a constant volley of signals to the thalamus. It is the role of the thalamus in this process, and the possibilities for intervention by the reticulothalamic axons, where Crick imagined the seeds of consciousness could be found.

When axons from layer VI of the cortex stimulate the thalamus, it sends back an immediate response, stimulating neurons in layer IV. All the calculations within a cortical module about whether or how to power up a pyramidal neuron and fire off a volley of signals are referred to the thalamus. The information returned by the thalamus is critical to whether the thought prepared within the cortical module is given a thumbs up or a thumbs down. Does the pyramidal motor neuron send a signal to the spinal cord? The thalamus helps decide. Every part of the cortex is in dialogue with its own specific, designated corner of the thalamus and it is the feedback from the thalamus, constructive or critical, that can either reinforce or, through lack of support, completely undermine the decision that a cortical module would like to make.

The way the thalamus responds to the queries from the cortex is shaped by experience, meaning and past rewards. This is where a rich pattern of learning is superimposed on the activity of Brodmann's areas to shape their activity. These memories are activated through other systems, and in particular two structures, the basal ganglia and the cerebellum, which also receive a copy of the deliberations by the cortex.

The basal ganglia sit just under the cortex and receive messages directly from neurons in layer VI. The more distant cerebellum channels the output of layer V pyramidal cell axons. The pyramidal cells of all the cortical areas that are not involved in movement extend axons towards the spinal cord, just like Betz cells, but terminate short of this destination, at a massive relay station in the brainstem called the pons. The pons diverts the reports from areas handling vision, hearing, language as well as movement and cognition up into the cerebellum, where the information is processed and fed back to the thalamus. The basal ganglia and cerebellum do different things with the information they receive before returning it to the cortex.

As brain users, we are barely aware of how the dialogue between the thalamus and cortex is adjusted to make changes in emphasis and meaning and timing. Perfecting a throw or the kick of a ball, or keeping the beat when we tap out a rhythm or dance: the feeling of 'being in the zone' is instinctive, mediated by the basal ganglia while the precision of action is finessed by the cerebellum. When either the basal ganglia or the cerebellum is damaged, the effects are far reaching across all areas of the cortex but are most obvious in the way we move. In Parkinson's disease, overactive basal ganglia shut down the responsiveness of the thalamus. It is difficult to start a movement, and to stop a movement once started. The decision-executing capacity of the cortex – its motivation to change – is sapped. By contrast, alcohol attacks cerebellar brain cells and the normally smooth and precise sequence of movements breaks down; we stumble, our speech is slurred.

Both the basal ganglia and the cerebellum are also needed for memories. The basal ganglia give the feeling of reward associated with doing something well for which you have trained or that you have experienced before. Without the cerebellum you simply cannot learn to play the violin or the piano. It not only helps to make movements precise, but also makes it possible to learn.

The actions of these structures are involuntary, associated with urges and reflexes, leading American neuroscientist Paul MacLean in the 1960s to claim they are part of a more ancient 'reptilian brain'. However, they are intimately involved in shaping complex thoughts and actions and we experience their actions even if they only come into play when the cortex is activated. But, this subliminal refinement is only part of the shadowland of the subconscious that Crick envisaged.

The way that the reticulothalamic nucleus would operate in Crick's theory was to define which of these cortical activities were brought sharply into focus and attended to and which were placed in the shadow. He called it a 'spotlight theory'.

Crick imagined our consciousness to be a shifting landscape of selected illumination where thoughts out of the spotlight carry on quietly not causing a disturbance. This is the result of inhibition by reticulothalamic neurons holding thalamic relays in check. The areas of the thalamus in the spotlight, able to operate in the glare of illumination, dominate our conscious selves, our attention and focus: our 'drawing eyes'.

In many ways, this chimes with my feeling of shifting conscious attention and, although I can never see inside your versions of consciousness, I assume (because you are a human reader of this chapter) that you may feel the same. But the idea that a spotlight theory based on a select group of brain calls might explain it all seemed highly improbable. To philosophers, it seemed ridiculously materialist; to psychologists, reductionist; to physicists, overly dependent on Newtonian thinking. Among neuroscientists, the appeal of emergent properties, as described by Penfield, seemed to be more suited to the vast complexity of the brain.

Undeterred by the criticism that his spotlight theory engendered from multiple angles, Crick moved on to another area of the brain. An island of cells called the claustrum became his later obsession, and he was writing about this structure in his hospital bed right up to the day he died in 2004. Once again, it was the architecture of the connections of its brain cells: the exchange of information between its neurons and every part of the cortex that excited Crick. The role of integrator and conductor of the audience of consciousness replaced the spotlight as a metaphor.

For both reticulothalamic neurons and the claustrum, a dependence on brain cell anatomy seemed to limit the reach of the theory. Animals without either a thalamus or a claustrum might be robbed of consciousness. This includes all invertebrates. And the claustrum is absent in fish, amphibians, reptiles and birds; all lack the kind of neural conductor that

Crick believed it represented. And although the claustrum can be found in most mammals, it is missing in marsupials where the pouch replaces the placenta. Is the kangaroo hopping about without conscious thought; is it a biological automaton? This seems unlikely.

However, it could also be seen as a liberating approach. It makes no judgements about which part of the brain is superior to the other. The teleological argument that consciousness must reside in the cortex, because that is what seems to distinguish thinking, feeling humans from other animals, is discarded. At the centre of consciousness are cells that can be conductors and operate spotlights; maybe different evolutionary strategies produced different forms of consciousness. Intelligent invertebrate creatures without either a thalamus or a claustrum – creatures such as an octopus – may have a different way of creating swathes of unconscious thoughts and a selective attention. If this is the case, then perhaps Crick was on the right track after all.

And there is something appealing about the theory of 'drawing eyes'. Maybe, just as the grand illusion that is our visual system hides the cracks, joins and holes that make up our imperfect whirring of neural machinery, perhaps we can only ever handle a very small part of multiple, simultaneous iterations of self that are held by the brain. The collective brain activity of billions of brain cells can be served up as a palatable story only by ignoring almost everything that they are doing to help our bodies survive. It is helpful to be directed towards the briefest of executive summaries, but we certainly do not need to know any of the details. Maybe, it really is that simple.

Cell 9

The Scheibel cell and the heterarchy

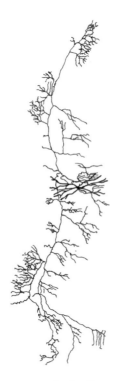

The giant reticular neuron in the hindbrain, which I name to myself the Scheibel cell. The dendrite sits in a contained space, with neighbouring dendritic trees (not shown) stacked up like poker chips. By contrast, the axon spreads far and wide into multiple territories, seemingly insinuating itself like a creeper or a vine throughout the brainstem.

Occasionally, just occasionally, as I was filling cells with dye, one after another during my doctorate, casually classifying them into *a*, *b* or *c*, I would come across an anomaly. It would be ten to twenty times larger than its neighbour, so rare that I had no idea what to make of it. It was so unexpected and unusual that I could not give it a name or fit it into any scheme and it sits still undocumented among the sheets of drawings that fill an old portfolio under my bed. These cells were so few and far between that they had to be left out of the story of my research. What else do you do with a single example of something that is an outlier – in this case, a brain cell whose function is unguessable?

Even as I started drawing and realised that its size required patching together of sheets of paper with Sellotape to make a canvas big enough to contain it, I knew this was never going to be talked about or worked into any theory of retinal ganglion cell function. Tracing a single cell across leagues of microscopic territory is quite a feat and I really, really wanted the cell to end. When a single dendrite began to span across a second sheet of A3 paper and threatened to breach a third it was already a hopeless cause.

For this reason, I had an acute understanding and respect for the reconstruction of each individual cell from a population of sprawling, enormous neurons that was traced by an academic husband and wife team in the 1950s.

Just after my PhD, I moved fields, changing disciplines to leave behind the retinal ganglion cells that I had been stalking for the previous five years. When you change your small focus of interest within science, you start again from scratch. You can read the textbooks and research the academic papers in the library, gaze at pictures that make little sense and try to get the feel of the territory, but still everything remains mysterious until you look at the thing itself down a microscope. I was in the uncertain phase of induction into a new part of the brain when I stumbled across the drawings of Arne and Madge Scheibel. My new field of study was the hindbrain (part of the brainstem not much wider than the spinal cord to which it connects), sitting just inside the skull and controlling everything from breathing to heart rate to the muscles that allow us to speak.

As students, we wanted to avoid thinking about the hindbrain at all. It seemed hideously complex, comprising interwoven strands of neurons, bundled together more or less as nuclei, with a cacophonous array of properties and functions. Clusters of cells control the muscles of the face and tongue, regulating all the subtleties of expression. Others, sitting to the side, are pacemakers for breathing, sensory cells for hearing or taste, further populations acting as regulators of heartbeat and breathing. Every species seemed to have its own variation of the arrangement of the component parts of the hindbrain around a central core that defied any logical architecture, or so it seemed. Understanding its structure seemed as complex as memorising the complete works of Shakespeare by heart. I avoided it.

However, in the later 1990s, the way in which the hindbrain developed in the embryo had suddenly become a dramatically simpler story. The catalyst was the advent of a new genetics that did two things. First, it showed that the same sets of genes were reused over and over in the animal kingdom, from insects to humans. With the sequencing of DNA, there was a realisation that genes were not only conserved but also arranged on chromosomes and controlled in similar ways in different organisms. Secondly, new cell staining techniques showed not only the structure of a neuron, but also whether a given gene was switched on or off within it. By mapping where in the brain specific forms of messenger ribonucleic acid (messenger RNA, the bridge between DNA and protein manufacture) were located, the activity of a gene could be logged under the microscope. This combination of advances had perhaps its most startling consequences on the understanding of the hindbrain.

It turned out that the dazzlingly complex brainstem in which the Scheibels' cell resided – that part of the brain whose anatomy you had to learn by rote rather than understand by the logic of its architecture – was incredibly simple in the early embryo. The hindbrain of all vertebrates was laid out in a series of eight segments that would later disappear, obscured by the mesh of overlying axons and clustered brain cell nuclei. Moreover, the segments were organised by the same genes that controlled the segmentation of the fly's body. Somehow the tools that sculpted the insect (Hox genes) had been redeployed or retained to make the hindbrains of fish, mice and man.

But what does the hindbrain do? In my myopic intensity of trying to understand one cell type for the previous five years, I simply had no idea what was going on in the rest of the brain. I was desperate to understand what I was doing in a new laboratory, anxious to be part of the conversation. The segmentation made sense. It seemed the hindbrain could be regarded as an ancient remnant of earlier brains. Making structures out of repeated compartments was something ancient and fly-like. But the function of the brainstem still seemed absurdly complex; like an abandoned garden, the elegant simplicity of the segment-like ground plan of this territory in the embryo was completely overgrown by a tangled mess of unruly brain cells. No sweeping, elegant, crystalline laminae of modular circuits as in the cortex. The hindbrain was a mess of small nuclei that controlled everything from basic life support to mating calls in birds, packed with a diverse array of neuroactive chemicals with no discernible pattern to their organisation.

The hindbrain had been regarded as an evolutionarily ancient structure since the early 1900s, but not because of its simple, early segmental form reminiscent of the body plan of the fly. This had been overlooked and it would be many years before genetics showed that the segments of insects and the human hindbrain were laid down by the same DNA codes. Instead, it was the tangled mess that stood in contrast to the pristine orderliness of the layered cortex, which spoke of primitive, messy connectivity. On top of this, the hindbrain seemed to harbour primal brain functions: breathing, heart rate, digestion, fight and flight. It was not the home of rarified cognition. Every sensation from inside and outside the body, from the depths of the gut to the sensation at our fingertips, is channelled through and deposits some information in the brainstem. Its seemingly impenetrable core was given the name 'the reticular formation'.

For the structures at the heart of the hindbrain, the naming as a reticulum seemed to me like an admission of defeat. This was a mess of neurons with connections to and from everywhere. It seemed the epitome of the tangled web of seemingly fused brain cells that the early anatomists had discovered with their tints and pigments in the mid-1800s. Everything else in the brain had elements of pattern and potential meaning. The reticular formation was the last stand of the impenetrable nerve mesh.

It was in the reticular formation that Arne and Madge Scheibel hauled in their enormous and seemingly inexplicably huge brain cell. I had come across a picture of it in a vintage book of conference proceedings – speeches and their responses – published in a hard-back volume in 1953. The Scheibels had used the black reaction, the Golgi stain, to uncover and reconstruct, piece by piece, a collection of neurons stretching over vast swathes of territory. I called it the 'Scheibel cell' in the laboratory and passed around the book with its page open at the picture of this enormous neuron.

The cell was vast, its axon filling the nooks and crevices of the brainstem and beyond, branching and changing shape, seeming to leak through the spaces to make sprawling tributary-like branches across a flood plain of brain tissue. The fingers of its spreading axon seemed totally different from branch to branch: dense as a frond of heather, articulated with short sprouting tendrils like a climbing ivy; or thin and fern-like, each twig budding off a main stem that forges a meandering path through the maze-like mesh of reticular core. This in itself seemed strange – any given neuron seems to have its own recognisable style of branching – but only as strange as the number of different parts of the brain it connected to.

The earliest foray into the reticular formation in the brainstem was made by a German neuroanatomist, Otto Deiters (1834–1863). Working almost twenty years before Golgi and Cajal started to see the structure of brain cells, Deiters teased individual neurons out of his preserved specimens using fine needles to pull the tissue apart. This seemed the only way that he could literally deconstruct the complexity of the brain and the cells emerged with at least some of their elaborate processes intact – enough to tell the difference between a single axon and protoplasmic processes (later recognised as dendrites). As these cells were dragged from the tissue, Deiters unknowingly also tore off the finest axon tips from other cells that were stuck to the dendrites of his partially isolated cells. Always reluctant to describe what he couldn't see, Deiters could not make a judgement call as to where one cell ended and another began – an ambiguity that was later seized upon as an argument that the net of neurons in the brainstem reticulum were fused into a continuous mesh. The core of the brainstem seemed stubbornly diffuse, and remained a rebuke to the theory of discrete neurons. Deiters' work was cut tragically short. After his father died, financial worries forced him into private medical practice. He caught typhus from a patient and died aged twenty-nine.[28, 3, 29]

Why did the Scheibels devote seven years of their lives to this part of the brain? The image I conjured in my mind's eye was of a grey-haired couple in the deep American Midwest, as far west and remote as Utah maybe. Somewhere with great scenery, very little in the way of distraction and endless time to contemplate the finer structure of the most complex tangle of cells in the brain. The opening paragraph of their 1958 chapter described their journey in the language of explorers of new lands rather than of scientists: 'In the Fall of 1950, we naively undertook the study of some of the fine structure of the brain stem . . . our hope has been to construct some kind of total image . . . we hope the data which we are about to report will be accepted in this spirit.'[30] How can we criticise this kind of endeavour? It immediately made me warm to Arne and Madge; I wanted to give them a hug.

The Scheibels' story attempted to put some order into a part of the brain that seemed to defy understanding. Apart from being a complex bundle of cells and their netted projections, the bewildering array of inputs into this area from all other parts of the brain defied an easy functional understanding of this core of the brainstem. Somehow, these inputs translate into a system of holistic regulation of body and mind in terms of muscle control to help you stand up straight, control your heart rate, blood pressure and respiration, maintain alertness. Long connections from the reticulum to the cortex can flood the cognitive brain with noradrenalin to stimulate or serotonin to alter mood.[31] The Scheibels' cell was somehow involved in both the rapid heart rate and shallow breathing of excitement, the drowsy contentment of sleep. These are the fundamental stages on which our neural systems play out their parts and shifting between them reconfigures all these interactions. This reticular neuron somehow embodied a stitching process that laced together parts of the central nervous system in complex and shifting ways.

The form of the Scheibel cell and the diverse and basic

life-supporting functions of the brain area in which it resides seemed so distant from the geometry of the cortex or the cerebellum. In contrast to the circuit-board-like precision of orderly layers and modular units, here was a messy, seemingly opportunistic cell, spreading like ivy over a wall with no clear plan. And yet the Scheibels' sprawling brain cells unwittingly became the unlikely obsession for one of the pioneers of computing and the substrate of a theory of value judgement in artificial intelligence.

At first glance, the scale and complexity of a single reticular cell offers little similarity to any of the geometry of any electrical circuit that might resemble a computer. However, the Scheibels made another important observation. Along with the almost preposterous, wandering branching and spread of the axons, able to thread their way through the reticulum, Arne and Madge realised that, in all their seven years of examination, every cell was similarly huge. They had never seen a single cell in the reticular formation with a short or even medium-sized axon. They were all giants.

In other words, the entire population was made of repeatedly interconnected neurons with no local circuits. And when Arne and Madge looked at the dendrites, another geometry emerged. Each dendritic tree was rather flat and arranged at right angles to the meandering axons. The dendrites spread across the reticulum at right angles to the up and down pathways of connections, sampling the information, like windmills in a breeze. In an architecture that reminded them of the precise right-angled organisation of Purkinje cells and their inputs in the cerebellum, it looked as if the dendrites of reticular neurons were stacked, like poker chips, in a series of segments.

Arne and Madge went further and began to speculate about how signals might jump between neighbouring axons, slowing down the progress of a signal and allowing it to be modified. They also speculated whether the inputs coming into every segment must carry all the different 'modalities' of information of the hindbrain: pain, touch, a signal from the cortex perhaps, information about blood pressure and carbon dioxide levels. All these strands of information would be passing through the dendrites in a breeze of data competing for the attention of the cell. When they drew their circuit, the stacked poker chips (each chip representing about 4,000 cells) looked a little like one of the 'lost' segments of the embryonic ground plan that preceded the reticular formation.

It was this poker-chip arrangement of dendrites, and the desire to reduce a complex geometry to something segmental and iterated, that attracted Warren McCulloch (1898–1969), one of the polymath figures of twentieth-century science, to delve deeply into the hindbrain.

I had come across McCulloch before I found out about the Scheibels and had no idea that he had been inspired by the work of Arne and Madge.[i] It was simply the title of one of his research papers that had fascinated me. 'What the frog's eye tells the frog's brain' by Lettvin, Maturana, McCulloch and Pitts, published in 1959, was such a provocative way to think of vision that, as a statement, it almost eclipses the substance of the article. The idea that the eye might be telling the brain a story felt like a reversal of my assumed hierarchy of brain function: the cortex sitting astride a sea of information and selecting and piecing together elements to create a logical picture. Here was a completely different proposition where the eye of any given animal could tell only one kind of narrative. We cannot escape the evolutionary disposition and biases of our senses.

As I delved further into Warren McCulloch, I found that his fame was far greater in computing than in neuroscience. Moreover, his unusual and original perspective on the 'frog's eye' as a narrator was as much about philosophy as science. In this provocative title, McCulloch was making a conscious reference to Immanuel Kant's proposition of a priori or innate notions of thought – a philosophical proposition dating from the 1700s.

At school, McCulloch had been destined to study theology, but he became increasingly interested in the philosophy of knowing: epistemology. At nineteen, he determined that his life's work would be to solve a riddle that he posed to himself in 1917: 'What is a number that a man may know it, and a man, that he may know a number?' First World War service in the US naval reserve derailed him from religion but his quest to understand the limits of human knowledge, which he saw as a question of analytical epistemology, had led him to Yale University to study philosophy and psychology.

The logical building blocks of the mind intrigued McCulloch, and at the start of the Second World War he became captivated by a new science of information theory, spurred on by the development of automated weapons. McCulloch, now a neurophysiologist and Head of Psychiatry at the University of Illinois, started conversations with Norbert Wiener, the founder of cybernetics, and collaborated with Walter Pitts (1923–1969), a young self-taught master of modular mathematics. Pitts was a teenage runaway who had been taken into the McCulloch family home at the age of sixteen and who, after reading *Principia Mathematica* at the age of twelve, had been exchanging letters with its author, Bertrand Russell.[ii] Inspired by psychiatry, taking the idealised brain cell as their model and Wiener's cybernetics as a guide, McCulloch and Pitts started to build a theoretical neural machine.

Their ideas focused on how feedback could be harnessed in a theoretical chain of neurons or 'psychons' to perform any logical mathematical operation. These ideas were combined into a 'logical calculus of ideas immanent in nervous activity' and published in 1943.[32] Typically for McCulloch, the paper was rich with philosophical allusions: the word 'immanence' recalled Kant's ideas about the revelation of innate knowledge, while psychon played on the concept of 'monads' as the units of a theory of mind put forward by Leibniz (1646–1716) a century before Kant.

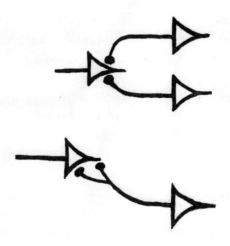

The graphical notation for psychons developed by McCulloch and Pitts representing neural building blocks of a logic calculus that could perform the operations of a Turing machine – the theoretical basis of modern computing.

Six years earlier, in a wartime role that would remain secret until the 1970s, the British mathematician and code-breaker Alan Turing had written a similar mathematical proof. His 'Turing machine' was a hypothetical device that could both read and write symbols on an infinitely long imaginary tape. In theory, it could execute any imagined mathematical instruction and it became the foundation for a code-breaking machine that cracked German naval signals. Moreover the Turing machine would be the basis of modern computing.

In their logical calculus, McCulloch and Pitts showed that simplified neurons, combined into feedback loops with the delays that might be expected in organic cells, could theoretically perform all the functions of a Turing machine. They had created the theoretical basis for an artificial brain made from synthetic neurons: it was the birth of artificial intelligence and machine learning.

With Pitts seconded to the Manhattan project and development of the atomic bomb, McCulloch continued to develop their concept of the neural net. Typical of his philosophical leaning, he wanted to explore how values might be communicated and used by his artificial neuron circuits to make choices. In 1945, he developed a theory of modular voting in a neural network that he called a 'heterarchy'. Each neural module in the heterarchy might take control of the circuit at any point and change its state.

The model explicitly harked back to his Officers Training Program in the Navy. McCulloch had been schooled in a key theory of naval warfare for ships of the line. In the heat of battle, with vessels spread across an expanse of ocean, command has to be able to shift seamlessly to the ship that has the most urgent or accurate information about the enemy's position and strength. Whatever the rank of the commanding officer, the warship in this position of informatic privilege takes control.

This control by 'redundant potential command' seemed an attractive model for decision-making that not only surpassed Wiener's cybernetics and feedback systems but also edged neural networks one step closer to a mathematical description of a living brain. However, for his model McCulloch still relied on symbolic psychons arranged in geometric loops that failed to resemble anything found so far within the brain. The theory seemed far removed from the messy reality of brain cells.

It was here that there was a remarkable meeting point between the complexity of Arne and Madge's cell and the pencil-drawn symbolic tools of McCulloch and Pitts. The Scheibels had embraced the complexity of natural form and intricately described one of the most complex of cell types in the most anarchic part of the brain. McCulloch and Pitts had reduced the complexity of the neuron to a psychon with a line for an axon and a triangle for a cell body.

Remember that the Scheibels had speculated that their cells were massively interconnected and that signals could navigate through the hindbrain along a number of different paths. Arne and Madge described the signals as 'tacking' their way up towards the cerebral cortex, like a boat sailing into the wind. I wonder if McCulloch, the ex-naval officer, was drawn to the nautical metaphor. He realised, twenty years after the publication of his heterarchy model, that in the giant Scheibel cell he had found the neuron he had been looking for.

In addition to the massive connectivity and the delays that were so important to the earliest models developed by McCulloch and Pitts, the poker-chip stacks (the segmentally arranged dendrites described by Arne and Madge) seemed to represent the ideal anatomical framework for a modular voting system of redundant potential command. Like warships at sea, McCulloch saw a command chain of modules, each capable of taking over the function priorities of the hindbrain: But what were the priorities they were choosing? The first line of his paper, published in 1969 with Bill Kilmer, summed up with characteristic bravado what McCulloch saw as fundamental choices that the Scheibels' cells were making in the brain: 'No animal can, for instance, fight, go to sleep, run away, and make love all at once.'[33]

The urgency of information dictates which module has control. McCulloch described a dolphin chasing its prey. Hunger drives the initial pursuit and this continues to be the global context in which all the brain's systems are operating until the dive becomes too long or deep and oxygen levels become critical. At this point, the switch in mode is sudden and complete – too quick for a hierarchical logic or feedback loops and too extensive to be controlled by anything other than a hugely interconnected but logically modular network. In McCulloch's proposition, this change in the fundamental mode of behaviour is the job of the Scheibels' cell. The most important signal controls the behaviour of the whole central nervous system regardless of competing sensations. Just like the first ship sighting an enemy taking control of the fleet.

Sleeping, fighting and making love are the series of incompatible choices in this theory. All segments, equally well connected to a huge range of inputs and talking to each other via vast axon networks, just as the Scheibels had themselves theorised, have an equal vote. But if one 'poker chip' urgently suggests sleep, the others fall instantaneously into agreement.

What had started as neural nets and Turing machines in the 1940s were now an artificial intelligence invested with self-regenerating behaviour and autonomy. A circuit that had the properties of a heterarchy could produce an artificial intelligence with the ability to take decisive and immediate action. Heterarchies might allow logical nets to control thinking and possibly feeling robots invested with appetites and urges. By marrying the Scheibels' brain cells, buried in the heart of the hindbrain, with the model he proposed in the 1940s, McCulloch linked his theory to the kinds of embodied changes that rule our everyday lives. It seemed his goal was as much to understand the poetry of the mind realised in the web of a neural net, as the mechanics of thought.[iii]

When Arne and Madge – in my mind, gnomic researchers in a quiet backwater – published their paper in the 1950s, it seems unlikely that they knew this would be the realisation of poetic dreams of the logic of mind of the already famous psychiatrist and polymath Warren McCulloch.

But as I dug deeper into the story of the Scheibels, my fantasy about them, which evolved from their disarming naivety in trying to tackle the monstrously complex reticular formation of the hindbrain, turned out to be wrong, or at least not entirely right. Neither were quiet Midwesterners. Arne Scheibel was a native New Yorker who spent his career in California as a neuroscientist and academic leader who continued to teach well into his eighties. His devotion to Madge was real. For fourteen years of illness before her early death, he rarely left their secluded California home, set within a rich botanical garden, surrounded by the entangled, sprawling branches of tropical trees and fantastically overgrown Scheibel bushes.

However, when I looked into Warren McCulloch, he proved to be exactly as I imagined. A rare television interview survives in which McCulloch, bearded and fiercely intellectual, is effortlessly dismissive of wrong-thinking, muddled and illogical ideas that mired his former profession of psychiatry. From classical scholar and apprentice theologian to head of the cybernetics laboratory at the Massachusetts Institute of Technology, McCulloch was true to the label of an eccentric, renaissance man: poet, psychologist, psychiatrist, neurophysiologist, neurosurgeon, philosopher, engineer and teacher.

He smokes continuously through the interview – a lanky body stretched on his overly small chair. It is easy to believe the claim that he sleeps, standing up, for only three hours a night, and easy to picture him swimming in his lake with some of his seventeen adopted children. He travels between cities in a travelling cape and hobnail boots, and lives off a diet of ice cream and whisky. He talks of his restless insomnia but lights up, with additional passion, when he talks about the scientists he has trained: his legacy, including seven professors in Holland. He died shortly after appearing on this early evening current affairs programme in 1967. As the interviewer explains, after the McCulloch conversation is aired, a bulging blood vessel is a ticking time bomb that Warren McCulloch would not discuss on television but that would shortly take his life. Walter Pitts, his amanuensis, died the same year at only forty-six years old.

This is an unfinished story. The reticular formation still feels mysterious and complicated. The proof of McCulloch's ideas has not yet been found. It requires an analysis of living networks during complex behaviours that is only now becoming possible within animals such as zebrafish. Psychons and heterarchy lie at the fringes of neuroscience. In much the same way, as well as being a pioneering figure in artificial intelligence, McCulloch as a neuroscientist may now be remembered better for a neat turn of phrase such as the story telling of a frog's eye.

However, I am drawn to the possibility that the segments from which the hindbrain forms – whose development I spent my time studying in my new laboratory, segments that disappear as the tangle of the reticulum emerges – are somehow important as organising modules. There are eight hindbrain segments, eight ships of the line, and these are conserved in every vertebrate from lamprey to human. Underneath the tangle of the overgrown garden of axons, massively interconnected in an almost impenetrable mess, first physically teased apart by Otto Deiters, then painstakingly reconstructed by Arne and Madge Scheibel, perhaps there is a simple plan. Eight segments with eight equal votes that switch us from neural context to neural context: we fight, we go to sleep, we run away, we make love.

Cell 10

The motor neuron, a final common pathway and Sherrington's ghost

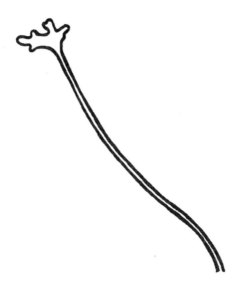

The symbolic neuron form adopted by Sherrington to explain the reflex in a few, select diagrams. The moss-like clubbed fingers represent the dendrites whereas the axon here is an open-ended tube.

'You've got to have a motor neuron. You can't not have a motor neuron. It's the "final common pathway".'

I'm sitting in my kitchen in east London with scientist friends and we are about to have an argument about what was to me the most utilitarian and dull cell – the one I had excluded from this book so far. The one I was about to reconsider.

Motor neurons filled me with a sense of something that I had left behind at school. A sense that the brain consisted of a single cell type, just as the skin has its epidermal cells and a carefully peeled translucent onion skin is made of miniature uniform tetrahedrons. Motor neurons were simply links between the brain and the body; they activate muscle and make us move. Somewhere in the brain there might be more cells, but the motor neuron (the Barker neuron) was the one that was always shown, clamped doggedly to a pink strand of muscle.

As I moved up the school and our representations of the brain became a little more sophisticated, the motor neuron became part of a key diagram – the reflex – depicting the arc of information from a receptor in the muscle via the spinal cord to the motor neuron and hence back again to the muscle. Sometimes this circuit was shown beside a disembodied knee and a little hammer to represent the patellar reflex. The motor neuron was the simple wire that connects the internal world with our body. The reflex was a simple and uninspiring window into what must be mysteries within the central nervous system. Maybe this early exposure explains the peculiar antipathy I felt to the motor neuron as a brain cell whose structure might tell an interesting story. It seemed like a dumb cell: the connector, a wire in a simple circuit.

So as I listened to the kitchen argument, the brightly coloured Barker neuron, the patella hammer and the circuit were running through my head: the stuff of six-year-olds, but the phrase 'the final common pathway' stuck. The story of the final common pathway is no less than a hunt for a physical home for the mind.

The motor neuron is not only the output of the central nervous system, but it is also our only way of interacting with the world, changing our environment. Picking up the coffee cup next to you, talking to a neighbour, winking to a friend, fighting global climate change – we do it all through these cells. The motor neuron is our means of communication, of expression and of exploring; it is our effector. Everything within the central nervous system must be channelled through the motor neuron population that stretches from the brainstem down the spinal cord, and whose axons are bundled together into paired nerves penetrating the body. These are some of the largest brain cells with axons that stretch from their cell bodies in the spinal cord to a muscle in the limb operating the most remote digit. At the end of each motor axon, a neuromuscular junction binds the nerve cell and the central nervous system to muscle. Electrical activity causes a muscle fibre to twitch and contract, pulling against the surrounding tissues, contorting our skin into a smile or swinging the masses of bone and muscle that pivot on smoothly articulated joints to let us run. Cell bodies of motor neurons are grouped into lozenges and columns, clustered together, their dendrites reaching out for contact with the circuitry of the brain.

Motor neurons are the most familiar of brain cells and most familiarly seen in the company of a sensory neuron in a reflex arc. They appear in our schoolbooks, pasted onto a diagram of a cross-section through a spinal cord – almost a perfect circle with an H-shaped core inside. Sticking out like arms from this circle, on either side, are two sets of nerves. In these diagrams, the sensory arm is always above and has a pronounced bulge where the cell bodies of sensory neurons in the dorsal root ganglion sit. These are drawn as a ball with a T-shaped addition representing the short pedicle and axon stretching from the skin or muscle, passing through the ganglion and continuing into the spinal cord.

Below this, in the drawing, the motor arm of the nerve also sticks outwards. The axon of the motor neuron runs through this nerve branch and its origin can be traced back to a ball, stripped of its dendrites, which represents the motor neuron cell body in the spinal cord. This was the standard two-dimensional diagram conceived by Waldeyer, who coined the phrase 'neuron doctrine' and supplicated by Barker who drew the first standard motor neuron. At school, it seemed very unexciting. Was this the mystery of the brain explained?

But although it appears simple, this standard diagram hides a complex past. It was the unlikely tool by which the synapse was imagined into existence in a step-by-step search for the illusive psyche by the British neuroscientist Charles Scott Sherrington (1857–1952).

When I had finished my undergraduate degree in Manchester, the studies for my doctorate took me to the University of Oxford and a department that had once been Sherrington's own. His face was one of the first I encountered as a young graduate student. My first degree in biology had little prepared me for entering what was hallowed ground – the home turf of a Nobel laureate[i] – and his legacy: his collection of papers and books, his box of slides, his name on a seminar room and, of course, his likeness. On the stairs in the entrance to the department was an oil painting of Sherrington with his younger collaborator, the Australian John Carew Eccles.

Something about the painting stuck with me: their moustaches and the peculiar wing-collar Victorian demeanour of Sherrington. I pitched him against the enigmatic, wildly imaginative Cajal, racing through countless nervous systems, piecing together the story of the brain from its elaborate architecture. By contrast, Sherrington seemed the epitome of the patrician British reserve – a physiologist who carefully measured muscle contractions in response to stimuli, calculating ratios of sensation to reaction. At a time when the black reaction was revealing the fabulous inner-cellular intricacies of the brain, he turned away from the brain cell in all but its most reduced and schematic form.

But the exploration of the motor neuron turns out to

be an exploration of the courteous and generous character of Sherrington, brought into sharp relief by his eventual meeting with Cajal. It is also a story of looking beyond the brain cell to its meaning in a circuit and building a logic of mind. Looking at this now, it is also an exploration of my own associations of school textbooks, assumptions about character and prejudices that can be followed back to that kitchen conversation.

Sherrington was born in Ipswich and at school became an avid scholar of Latin and Greek and a poet. Despite his devotion to classical studies, he nevertheless chose to train as a doctor at St Thomas' Hospital, London, before transferring to Cambridge University, maintaining a passion for writing a poetry of elaborate language – words such as 'assoiled', 'meseemed' and 'reft' – that would seep into his scientific writing. He was drawn into a world of experimental physiology and experiments on the localisation of function in the brain, working first in Strasbourg and then Berlin before returning to St Thomas' and Cambridge. In 1885, a cholera outbreak in Spain brought Sherrington and a young Santiago Ramón y Cajal to Toledo and Zaragossa at the same time, although the two were not destined to meet for another nine years.

On his return to England, Sherrington set about performing a systematic exploration of the brain. However, unlike Cajal, there was no need to look at nerve cell structure. Although Sherrington was skilled with the microscope, the cellular basis of the brain was not the focus of his interest. He set out with an idea that if he could take the reflex arc and understand how it was modified in the context of the whole animal, he could begin to explore the brain beyond the reflex. The same generic circuit diagram of Waldeyer and Barker could become a key to unlock hidden and as yet invisible complex reflexes. To remove as much distraction as possible, it seemed to me as if Sherrington mentally pruned the dendrites of the motor neuron and converted the Barker neuron into a diagrammatic symbol.

With the reflex arc reduced to a series of symbolic actors, Sherrington began to test the logic of this diagram by examining the operation of the circuit in the whole animal. Crucial to this approach was the idea that the output of the final common pathway was the sum of whatever came in by way of stimulus plus the contribution of the black box of the brain. Changing the conditions in a logical way would start to reveal the workings of the black box. Brain cells were essential but only as algebra. The motor neuron, or FC (final common), was the answer to an equation whose unknown variables (a, b, c etc.) could be deduced by systematically changing the experiment.[ii]

Piece by piece, with each set of the experiments, the arrangements of symbolic neurons began to produce predictable results. For the first time, Sherrington could identify the properties of the join between nerve cells and give a name to it: the 'synapse'. It would be many years before the synapse could be seen using an electron microscope, but Sherrington did not need to visualise the miniscule gaps between adjacent cells; he reasoned that the communication across a membrane-to-membrane interface between brain cells had to have one-way or 'rectifying' properties that allowed information to be passed in only one direction. Without seeing something that would remain invisible for another fifty years, Sherrington imagined an explanation at a molecular scale simply by his measurements of experimental muscle contraction.

Sherrington summarised a huge body of his work in a single volume, *The Integrative Action of the Nervous System*.[34] It is not a book that can be browsed in the same way as Cajal's two-volume *Histology of the Nervous System* with its illustrations on every page decorating the text like an illuminated manuscript. In Sherrington's *Nervous System*, there are four diagrams of ball-and-stick neuron circuits and eighty-five illustrations, the majority of which are traces of muscle contractions.

The contrast between these different treatises on the brain is a contest between the word and the image as a form of argument. The brain cell still lies at the core of Sherrington's work but its structure is not shown, except stripped back to what is necessary to illustrate the text. What he omits in terms of the beauty of illustration is replaced by a gradual and compelling argument that tackles that most elusive of neural concepts, the psyche. As Sherrington traces out the gradual construction of complex reflexes, it feels like the hunt for an elusive quarry which dodges the searchlight, until finally Sherrington has it cornered by physiology.

His reasoning still holds up as an exercise in logic. The final common pathway is the product of the integration of everything that goes on between sensation entering the body and the motor neuron activating a muscle. Sensors on the skin, or within a muscle, receive direct input from physical stimuli and activate local responses: a stretched ligament causes your knee to jerk, a cold surface makes you pull your finger sharply away. However, these can be inhibited or overcome by more urgent commands, as Sherrington could demonstrate: you can pick up an ice cube with your fingers and extinguish the reflex without thinking twice. The ability to override a reflex demonstrated the existence of something extra – circuits within the brain beyond the simple reflex arc.

Working upwards from the spinal cord towards the brain, Sherrington deconstructed the roles of the receptors of the most immediate sensations, on the skin and in ligaments, and then of distant senses – sound and vision. Importantly, this second group of 'exteroceptors' tells the brain not only about events that do not directly touch us but also, Sherrington reasoned, about what may be about to happen. This allows for the generation of an association between a stimulus and the possibility of direct physical interaction. You see a wall ahead and sense there is a potential collision. The collision takes place and the association between the signals from the exteroceptors and sensors on the body is remembered. At one end of the spectrum, learning by association allows bad things to be avoided. But at the opposite pole of experience, the exteroceptors and the displacement in time between a distant object and its consummation in some form allows expectation. Sherrington called this new integrative property 'conation' – purpose or desire. I see or hear something that would be beneficial, be it sustenance or behavioural reinforcement: a social contact, a stroke, a kiss. The space between detection and the possibility of consummation creates room for motivation, a reason to act. Suddenly the transition from spinal cord to brain becomes the transition from mechanical reflex to planning, thought and emotions.

Sherrington saw the evolution of exteroceptors as critically linked to the development of locomotion. The placement of the exteroceptors at the front of the animal, the predominant direction of movement, was an essential driver of the development and evolution of a head, the brain and the origins of motivation.

Sherrington seized on a natural proof of the link between conation, the head and senses. The sea squirt is an anemone-like filter-feeding sac with a nervous system that is little more than a net of reflexively responding electrical fibres with no central organising head. But as a young animal, the sea squirt (or ascidian) larva is a free-living creature with exteroceptors in its head, a mobile tail and a primitive spinal cord called the notochord. Not only did the head evolve to concentrate our senses around the need for sustenance and a drive to move, but when an animal loses its locomotion, the head and nervous system regress, confirming this correlation for Sherrington.

Sherrington described the stimulation of the distance receptor as 'pre-current'. In other words it was informing the brain of something that could happen to 'current' receptors such as those on the skin in the future. The gap before that might take place was the space for learning and association to come into play. Most importantly, by extrapolating from these basic behaviours, Sherrington created a theoretical space in which the mind could begin to take shape.[iii]

Sherrington was not stating that eyes and ears see into the future. Their responses are every bit as current as a touch or a pinch. However, it was the interval between anticipation and effect – the pre-current sensation of a possibility and current realisation of its occurrence – that had allowed the mind to emerge. For Sherrington, it also set its boundaries. Not only might it mean that the adult sea squirt has literally 'lost its mind' by abandoning pre-current sensations, but it also meant that the mind's reach was defined by sensation. In his typically florid writing style, the act of eating becomes the action by which:

> Into that sequestered nook the organism by appropriate reactions gathers morsels of environmental material whence by chemical action and by absorption it draws nutriment.[iv]

And in the act of swallowing, Sherrington saw one of the key boundaries of the conscious mind: the point where attention to food is given up to the relatively vague and imprecise sensations of digestive system 'interceptors'.

Without offering a definition of the mind, Sherrington had attempted to define the boundaries of the terrain in which it must exist – between anticipation and summation, the distant detection and the reflex response. He traced the origin of the space it inhabits in evolution and defined how the pre-current sensations of sound, sight and smell conjure up a world of possibilities for the mind to play with. The space in between is a space for desire, fear, love, hate. Sherrington's version of the psyche maps a landscape of affordances, which gives way, resists or responds to our actions mediated by that final common pathway, the motor neuron.

If Sherrington's model holds true, then perhaps it also allows us to peer into our own, possibly near, future. What if the space between our sensation and our motor neurons – the final common pathway – becomes stretched by our evolving or artificially enhanced senses? We can extend by proxy the range to our pre-current receptors using technology to see a different spectrum of colour, sense heat at a distance, see through solid objects, be aware of the movement of everyone within a mile radius. Arguably technology has already had an effect on the way we think and feel. But what if we are plugged directly into these new sensors so that they integrate with the delicate circuitry of our brain? How would an altered exteroception change the fabric of our mind? In Sherrington's model, the dimensions in which our mind is free to develop and explore would be far larger, more spacious and a powerful engine for evolution.

In my imagination I had pitched Sherrington, who seemed to find little interest in images of the neuron, against Cajal, who celebrated in its elaborate diversity. But when they eventually met, there was both respect and what seemed to be an unlikely but firm and affectionate bond. A decade after their paths almost crossed during the cholera epidemic, Sherrington invited Cajal to give the 1894 Croonian Lecture at the Royal Society. Sherrington, the Victorian classical scholar and Cambridge don, was struck by Cajal's raw energy and excitement: a 'peasant genius'. He stayed in the Sherringtons' home, baffling hosts and their neighbours as he daily hung his bedclothes out of the window to air, heedless of British weather. On the day he was to receive an honorary doctorate from Cambridge University, he accidentally caught an earlier train from London and found no one to meet him at his destination and had no idea where to go. Not speaking a word of English, he strolled into town to explore. He paused to sketch the façade of Emmanuel College but stood in the middle of the road to do so, disrupting the traffic. Unable to be understood or to understand, he attracted the attention of the police. He missed the lunch in celebration of his visit, but did eventually receive his honorary degree, only after a worried Sherrington had searched the town and eventually contacted the local constabulary.

One sharp difference between Sherrington and Cajal was their perspectives on the mind and spirit. Sherrington's work had been a careful calibration of the dimensions of the black box in which such things could exist. His search had, perhaps by chance, come up against the limits of the psyche, a word that encompasses the mind, but also the spirit and the soul. I wonder whether Sherrington, the poet, felt a conflict between his empathetic understanding of the soul and his scientist's drive to contain and measure it. Sherrington was dismayed that Cajal could breezily accept that the psyche was nothing more than the physical and chemical properties of cells within the brain. Speculation was almost a fruitless exercise – mind and spirit emerged from and were entirely found within the workings of brain cells. This was something that Sherrington found hard to accept. Cajal's perspective, rooted in the world of the neuron and focused on the material components of the brain, left little room for what Sherrington described as the 'zest of the waking day'.

Perhaps Sherrington, steeped in classical history and deeply in love with a language of soulful expression, had come as close to defining the psyche as he could bear to. His analytical approach to the reflex, synapse, receptor, the exteroceptor defined the limits of free will. Sherrington brought science face to face with poetry, the contradictory passions that had defined his own life. He had cut and sliced up the nature of interaction between the outside and inside world until left with an irreducible space, small but well defined, where the soul, if it is truly part of the physical property of the mind, must exist. At this point, Cajal simply chose to shrug and look away. The argument was fruitless. But for Sherrington, the idea that there was no ghost in the machine – that it was simply a mix of chemicals, electrical impulses and the synapse that he himself had invented – denied the very poetry of life.

Cell 10½

*The giant axon and
the little yellow spot*

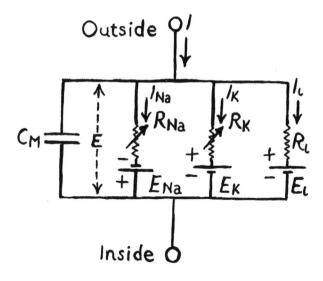

*The abstraction of neuronal form into a circuit diagram by Hodgkin and
Huxley is the ultimate abstraction of the neuron: from connector in a
network to computational device in its own right.*

As much as the story of the brain is the story of the brain cell, the neuron all but disappeared from swathes of neuroscience in the latter half of the twentieth century. The reason was that the brain cell, in all its elaborate beauty, had been captured, completely and comprehensively, within a single mathematical equation. It was transformed into an electrical diagram, the kind of circuit board that we might construct at school with batteries, rheostats and light bulbs. Most importantly, the circuit board diagram was sufficiently powerful to explain the chemistry and physics of how brain cells communicate – the all-important substrate of thought itself. However, this was not a model of a whole brain cell but of only one part: its membrane. The story of the half a brain cell is the tale of the exploration of the skin of a neuron using fragments of the largest of all axons, discovered in 1909 in the common squid by Leonard Worcester Williams (1875–1912).

Theoretical models are a special thing in science that are used in different ways. They can be a blackboard scribble on which ideas are tested, a physical structure like the models of DNA made by Crick and Watson. Some have a practical purpose to test a hypothesis and others express a theory in its most elegant form. If a model survives being twisted and examined from every angle, it gains currency and takes on a life of its own. It becomes almost independent of its creators as it is copied, passed on, printed again, examined in classrooms, or used as a roadmap in the lab. In some ways, the model breaking free from its creator, becoming traded and gifted, resembles the trajectory of a successful work of art, created in the studio, but then outliving its creator to pursue an independent destiny in a gallery or museum. The success of a model depends on its endorsement, its ability to communicate and in some cases its capacity to open doors to a new way of looking at the world. The electrical model of the brain cell is one of these. It is a theory that survives intact at the heart of a multitude of more complex models and computer simulations – a lens through which the brain cell is reduced to the flow of ions in either direction in and out of a cell.

The nerve cell membrane occupies a special place in my life. It was my foe in the lab. My constant battle with the microscopically thin veil of fat defined success and failure of my research for my doctorate. I was trying to push a needle-sharp piece of glass into a cell. The flexible layers of lipids, only two molecules thick, that make up the membrane could seem as impenetrable as a thick sheet of India rubber.

A strange thing happens when you handle cells and tissue under a microscope. You begin to feel the forces and objects as a physical sensation even though these entities are too small to grasp or feel. Distances are measured in a few thousandths of a millimetre with tools that vanish to thin points that almost disappear under the microscope lens. Experimenters use eyelashes to slice up parcels of tissue from frogs' eggs in just the same way as in the 1920s. And even though the forces are too small to register at your fingertips, when you see a cell cut by an eyelash or chopped by a filament of wire under the microscope, you feel and sense these movements. I can remember the perspiration building on my forehead as I attempted to make a cut into a thin sheet of tissue, one tenth of a millimetre across, with a piece of sharpened tungsten wire too thin to see. There is no real, tangible resistance transmitted along the tungsten, into the glass rod to which it was glued, to my hands poised about the petri dish. But it felt as impenetrable and tough as leather, although the slightest involuntary muscle twitch would have destroyed it utterly. I avoided coffee on the day I was dissecting to reduce the microscopic tremors in my hands that would rip the tissue to pieces.

The glass tube of a micropipette, sharpened to a point, is one step further removed from the senses because it is held by an assembly of levers, springs and calibrated dials. But still its movement becomes part of my movements. As I sit at the microscope the sharpened glass tube, a fraction of a millimetre in diameter and invisibly fine at its tip, is being driven by a heavy Huxley manipulator named after its inventor.

My own Huxley manipulator is lemon yellow and very cool to the touch, a dense block of precision parts. Putting my nose close to it, I can smell the precision in the machine oil. Three chunky dials can be rotated to move the tip of the glass tube smoothly in three dimensions, one-thousandth of a millimetre per click. The movement of the dials, conveyed by a system of rods, translates the twist of a hand into the smallest movement at the tip of the glass. After a week or two, the movements required to swing the glass tip under the microscope and gently approach the cell become second nature.

I feel as if I'm throwing this glass rod across the surface of the brain, stopping just in time as the tip grazes the surface of a sheet of neurons.

As I touch the surface with the tip of the glass, the rotation of the dials gets heavier, more difficult. Seeing the tip advance by fractions of a millimetre, the wavering tone from the amplifier suddenly dips as the open end of the glass nudges up against the membrane of the neuron.

The membrane feels tough and bends as I push forward but doesn't give. I don't want to push the whole cell out of place. The loosely anchored dendrites are flexible but delicate. One break and the neurons would never hold the dye that I was about to pump in. It would just flood out. I feel that resistance as the neuron is gently displaced, but not punctured by its tip. The final tap, infinitesimally small, feels like puncturing a balloon and bright yellow dye floods into the cell.

This sensation of resistance, the pressure and tension of pushing against a flexible rubber ball that just won't puncture, is all illusion. But it is burned into the muscle memory of my body. It still makes me tense up. The sense of frustration as the narrow glass tip slips and slides past its target or ruptures a cell and the sight of precious yellow dye spilling like mist over the landscape under my microscope. Then the exultation when the pipette makes a clean stab and the yellow dye, contained and concentrated, picks out the delicate shape of a brain cell. The shape of the brain cell is the shape of its cell membrane and, as Huxley discovered, it is the cell membrane that allows the neuron to speak.

Andrew Huxley (1917–2012), the engineer who designed my manipulator, was an experimental tinkerer – a neuroscientist who, in my imagination, valued the perfection of the tools of experimentation almost as much as its outcome.[i] His name lives on in the machines he designed for use in the laboratory but moreover in his work on the mathematical description of the neuron with Alan Hodgkin (1914–1998) – the circuit board diagram of capacitors, resistors and rheostats – that won them both the Nobel Prize in Physiology or Medicine.

They appear on the cover of the 1963 Nobel Prize brochure in a picture entitled 'Nerve Cell Enigma Solved'. It stages an incongruous assembly of objects relating to their careers. Against a mustard background, two middle-aged men pose in matching waistcoats and ties, sleeves rolled up, ready to get down to work on some serious science. Andrew Huxley pauses over a small microscope, adjusting controls. Alan Hodgkin peers over the top of the small stack of modular electronics, facing away from him. The imaginary object of the experiment sits on a small microscope linked by wires to an amplifier that is attached to an oscilloscope – a device that converts a change in voltage into a trace on a small round screen. The colours are intense and lurid. The whole scene is framed by a circular olive-green border. In front of them, in the foreground, is an enormous, bright red lobster.

But what was this enigma, and how had they solved it? Hodgkin and Huxley had successfully deconstructed the neuron to answer a fundamental question: how are rapid signals passed between brain cells and generated within them? The answer lay at the surface of the brain cell. They needed to dismantle the neuron into its component parts, both conceptually and physically. And so they chose an animal to study whose neurons were large enough to cut up, squeeze, suspend and manipulate without destroying their function. By doing this, they cast a different vision of the brain cell: a collection of idealised geometries whose surfaces formed the tabletop for chemical reactions and whose sinuous form became elevated, or reduced, to a mathematical equation.

The bright red lobster in the Nobel picture is its most incongruous feature. I can only imagine that it happened to be readily to hand when the photographer learned that the scientists worked on animals without backbones. Perhaps there was a hurried pre-shoot visit to the local deli counter to retrieve a cooked lobster. However, Hodgkin and Huxley's discoveries, and subsequent Nobel Prize, came from the meticulous chopping and dissecting of a different, perhaps less photogenic, invertebrate: the long-finned squid, *Loligo forbesii*.

Loligo is a creature that can reach almost a metre long, with brain cells buried under its tough spear-shaped mantle that send out axons so large that for many years they were thought to be circulatory vessels of some kind and not part of the nervous system. In his 1909 monograph, Leonard Williams marvelled at their size, so large that they might easily be overlooked as neurons and it was 'well nigh impossible' to believe that fibres that disappeared into the mantle were axons. They reminded him of the giant nerve fibres found in fish that belong to Mauthner cells. Triggering a Mauthner cell generates a dramatic escape response that contorts the body and drives the fish away from danger. In the squid, he could not see which part of the body the axons were connected to but his guess that they might have a similar function proved to be correct. The giant axons that he had discovered can trigger a powerful jet propulsion that propels a squid to safety.

Williams was to die young in a freak elevator accident

at Harvard University and his observations, buried in his description of the anatomy of *Loligo*, were seemingly forgotten. Twenty years after his death, the rediscovery of these giant axons, almost half a millimetre in diameter, gave scientists a brain cell that, for the first time, they could dissect into its various parts. The axon was large enough to be picked up with a pair of tweezers – large enough to roll flat, reinflate and slide over a fine glass tube.

And this is exactly what Huxley and Hodgkin did. By hanging the dissected axon in a jar of sea water and using two small mirrors at right angles, they guided the glass into the tube of axon. They used the glass tube as an 'electrode' and by measuring the difference in charge with this, inside the membranous tube, and a wire dipped into the surrounding bath of cold sea water, they could see the voltage difference between the inside and outside of the axon. The further the glass rod was inserted, the greater this became, until it sta-bilised at -55 mV.

This constant difference between the inside and outside of the membrane is now known as the resting potential. 'Potential' because, in the right circumstances, the charged ions could flood across the membrane to create an electrical current. And 'resting' because of what Hodgkin and Huxley did next. They applied a current to the cut end of the axon and discovered that at a certain threshold the membrane suddenly took on a life of its own. In place of timid waves of electricity, giant pulses of energy suddenly shot along the axon. The resting membrane jumped from negative to positive and back to negative again almost instantaneously. Each pulse had the same height and, crucially, whatever the length of the axon, the pulse of electricity (an 'action' potential) never decayed.

The wave of electrical excitation was self-regenerating. Here was a basis for neural communication over long distances using pulses of electricity that could travel any distance at terrific speeds. From there, it was a natural step to ask whether information might be coded in the frequency of the pulses. If so, this could be a basis for a language of neuron communication. And so, in 1939, Hodgkin and Huxley published the first ever recording of an action potential – in the squid's giant axon, a half a cell suspended in a jar of sea water.

The resilience of the giant axon to handling, cutting, cleaning and suspending allowed a host of experiments in the following decade. The duo had established that it was the surface of the axon that was important for transmitting action potentials; however, the circuit diagram was not finalised until 1952. By this stage, they had adapted their glass rod to measure the flow of charged ions, through what turned out to be tiny channels in the membrane. What made the action potential possible was that each electrical stimulus forced tiny pores to open transiently, allowing ions to flood across the membrane. This current stimulated the next patch of membrane, and so on, in a chain reaction that carried the pulse along the axon.

All these subsequent discoveries relied on that first stable resting potential that Hodgkin and Huxley had observed as they slid the glass rod into the suspended sheath of the giant axon. It turned out that this difference in voltage across the membrane relies on an active and hugely energy-intensive one-way pumping of positively charged sodium ions from the inside to the outside of the cell. Sixty per cent of our brain's energy is used in this one task of maintaining the membrane's lop-sided polarity.

Perhaps the strangest experiments came ten years later, when the entire contents of the axon (its axoplasm) was rolled out as a jelly into the dish using a handheld cylinder on an axle. Somehow, this resembles in miniature the garden roller that makes cricket pitches and lawn tennis courts flat – something that, perhaps, was not incidental. I can almost imagine the inspiration for the handheld lawn roller in the immaculate lawns of a Cambridge college. Using the roller to squeeze out the contents of the axon allowed experimenters to replace its contents with different solutions with different concentrations of ions.

This final experiment had entirely deconstructed the brain cell. Gone were its cytoplasm, the cell body, dendrites and cytoskeleton to leave nothing but the membrane itself – the skin of the neuron. Within the two layers of sandwiched lipids, speckled with channels and pumps that regulate the passage of ions, is all the machinery that is sufficient for communicating information and making axon potentials. The membrane was the engine of cell communication. The half a brain cell had solved the enigma of how brain cells talk to each other.

But how did squid anatomy become the solution to the problem of neural communication in the first place? The story of the giant axon experiments started a decade earlier in the Bay of Naples at the Stazione Zoologica marine biology research institute where two young scientists, Enrico Sereni (1900–1931),[ii, 35] and John Zachary 'JZ' Young (1907–1997), were studying the nervous system of cephalopods. They had become fascinated by a curious yellow spot on the surface of the head of the squid's cousin, the evolutionarily sophisticated and fiercely intelligent octopus. The yellow pigmented gland, no bigger than a pinhead, sits just above the 'epistellar' ganglion of the octopus, and Sereni and Young were determined to discover its function.

Although similar to the squid in many ways, the octopus is a very different beast. Its brain is larger and more consolidated. In many animals without backbones, the function of the central nervous system is spread between ganglia that are distributed through bodies that are often segmented. Not so in the octopus, which has central brain lobes regulating coordinated locomotion, eye movements and colour changes. Two central lobes defy easy characterisation with functions that are abstract enough to suggest a sophisticated intelligence. Unlike the squid, the arms of the octopus are packed full of nerves rather than muscle alone and perform motor movements with huge degrees of freedom while accumulating a mass of sensory information. The overall behaviour of the octopus is complex, intelligent and conscious. With simple logic, Sereni and Young first decided to remove the yellow spot, in a rapid and painless surgery under anaesthetic. The results were poignant and this largely forgotten episode may well have shaped JZ Young's attitude towards the octopus and cemented its status as an intelligent and conscious being.

Despite this apparent brutality, removing part of the brain to understand its function seemed a reasonable idea in the 1930s. The discoveries of brain regionalisation in the human cortex gave hope that careful surgery might help patients suffering from a range of mental health problems. At around the time that Sereni and Young were researching in Naples, Egas Moniz (1874–1955), a Portuguese surgeon, started to perform frontal leucotomies or lobotomies that severed the connections to and from the front of the brain. Patients who suffered from what were characterised as behavioural disorders from depression or uncontrolled aggression to what was perhaps simply teenage rebellion seemed to be cured. The lobotomy rapidly became a standard treatment and Moniz received a Nobel Prize in 1949.

However, disquiet began to grow in the 1940s about the effects of this radical psychosurgery. Patients were relieved of the problems that had recommended them for surgery but would be rendered listless, apathetic, lacking in drive or interest or at worse reduced to the behavioural capacity of a toddler. This was the fate of Rosemary Kennedy, JFK's 'forgotten' sister who was operated on at the age of twenty-three, following a rebellious adolescence, and remained institutionalised for the rest of her life. The target of the lobotomy was the prefrontal cortex which seemed to Moniz to be a source of all the distress in patients with perceived personality disorder. However, it is also the seat of judgement and decision-making. Its destruction led to a profound and irreversible change in personality. By the late 1960s, after tens of thousands of operations, the lobotomy was shunned.

The removal of the tiny epistellar body – the yellow dot – had a remarkable and profound effect in Sereni and Young's octopus patients. The surgery appeared to have the same effect as a lobotomy in humans. The animals hung from the side of the tank with limp arms. Instead of moving about actively, they remained attached to the sides, Young wrote, giving a striking picture of depression. They were emotionally lacklustre and listless, and their characteristic colour changes were muted. We now know that octopuses are sensitive to their environments; they recognise their favourite human researchers and fall into that intriguing cluster of creatures that can use tools. But after surgery, their playfulness and interest in the world around them disappeared.

Young and Sereni changed course, reckoning that the yellow spot might be a remnant of the photoreceptor system from a more primitive, squid-like ancestor. They turned to the squid for answers, rediscovering that, as Williams had found before, a collection of giant axons that had long since disappeared through the evolutionary history of the octopus, emerged from the epistellar ganglion and disappeared into the mantle. Young and Sereni found that a mixture of different sizes of axons from the epistellar ganglion fed into the powerful muscles that provide the squid with its jet-propulsion system. The largest of the collection of fibres, the giant axon, fed the most distant muscles – an important fact because, as measured much later by Young, larger axons carried signals much quicker than smaller ones. This meant that a single stimulus would send a signal that arrived at all the muscles both distant and close at the same time, generating a coordinated jet of water and a cloud of ink. They had found in giant axons what Williams had predicted in 1909: the basis of an escape response.

However, the function of the little yellow spot in the octopus – the starting point for Young and Sereni and the ultimate origin of Hodgkin and Huxley's brain cell model – remains a mystery. Although the yellow epistellar body never regenerated in their experiments, the octopus seemed largely to recover after a week or so. Like human lobotomy patients, I wonder whether their recovery was all that it seemed. Did this poignant and largely forgotten episode shape Young's attitude towards the octopus? Not only was its behaviour complex and intelligent, but individuals had a personality that could be radically altered by his inadvertent psychosurgery. After the death of Sereni, a committed anti-Fascist, in mysterious circumstances, Young returned to England and his studies on the octopus brain. But he also became a powerful advocate for the octopus as a creature of special status among animals without backbones. It remains the only invertebrate protected from unlicensed experimentation by law in the United Kingdom.

The story of the squid giant axon that could be divided up, squeezed, rolled and stimulated in a dish has an ironic twist. It is not, as first thought, a single brain cell at all and, according to a contemporary account, Young knew this. The clue comes in an account by Rainer 'Ray' Guillery (1929–2017), a professor of anatomy at Oxford of whom I was in awe as a PhD student, in an article that highlighted the contribution of his great-grandfather's younger brother, Otto Deiters, to the neuron doctrine.[iii] Ray had completed his PhD in 1954 in a University College London department headed by JZ Young, and had always been puzzled by an incident concerning a lecture by a visiting scientist. An anatomist from Bonn had given a seminar and described a hypothesis that there could be, in certain circumstances, a fusion of nerve cells. This was evidence he believed that contradicted the nerve cell doctrine of Cajal, the central tenet of modern neuroscience. The idea of fusion or 'anastomoses' harked back to the early days of the reticulum and the nerve net. Ray was completely taken aback by the violence of consternation from a normally mild JZ Young. And yet this fusion was something that Young had seen for himself, within the squid epistellar ganglion.

Feeling like I had stumbled onto a hidden family secret, and following Ray's clues, I searched through Young's original papers on the squid giant axon, written just before the Second World War. In almost an offhand comment, Young paused to speculate on the origin of the giant nerve cell itself. The axon was so large – huge in fact – that at first it seemed it could not be nervous tissue but some kind of secretory capillary. But where was the cell body? As Young traced the root back to its origin, it revealed not a giant cell body, as he expected, but a tube that was fed by anything from 800 to 1,500 separate cells joined together in a single fused community. The squid giant axon that would unlock the secrets of how information was transmitted in the neuron was not a cell at all. It was a syncytium, a nerve mesh, the proof of a theory that had challenged the neuron doctrine at its inception in the late 1800s. Here was a single axon formed of a thousand cells.

The existence of cell fusions, not uncommon in invertebrates but largely overlooked by many neuroscientists, does not challenge the idea that the brain is made of cells. But it does remind us always to look again. Even the most resilient of models, like the neuron diagram of Hodgkin and Huxley – founded not in an analysis of a single enormous cell, but the fusion of a colony of neurons – can always be approached with a healthy scepticism. A second look.

Epilogue

The storytelling brain

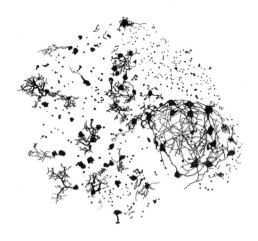

The fragments and scattered cells of a Golgi-stained rat cerebellum drawn through a camera lucida. On the dusty shelf and brought out occasionally for a demonstration, this now precious glass slide is rarely explored. This scene took some hours to draw over the course of an evening. I tried to capture every detail of a view that would have confronted Santiago Ramón y Cajal when he first encountered Golgi's revolutionary technique. I forced myself to focus on the things I would ignore: the fragments of cell body lacking dendrites or axons and a myriad of small dots – what are they? Tiny cells or random condensations of black reaction? I do not know. Normally, my pen would skip over these inconvenient inclusions. I would concentrate on the scattered Purkinje cells and a swirling nucleus of cerebellar output neurons that jump off the page to my eyes, perhaps arranging them into a more orderly scene in a semi-diagram. Do you see these cells? Easy when you know what to look for, but what if this were the first time they have ever been made visible. Where do you look? What do you look for?

Doing science is rather like peering through a small gap in a fence at a huge landscape beyond. As you scan to a new feature of interest, the trees and hills you were just looking at disappear. Look back again and the view you remembered is totally different. You will never be able to scale the fence. Everything is a tantalising glimpse of an unreachable whole.

A hundred scientists looking through different cracks, eyeholes, chinks, see a different view. Comparing what we see becomes the gossip and chatter at the end of the day. We build a story and feel it's satisfying enough to publish in an anthology. We are passionate about our version of the tale, but others disagree and the rumble of voices carries on. Some of us are more patient and cautious in extrapolating a sense of what the landscape holds from such a narrow field of view. The crack in the fence is restricted and none of it adds up in a satisfactory way. We work as groups to build our sense of reassurance. Others are more confident; everything fits as part of a coherent model in their minds. And if it doesn't, the model can change. There are points of agreement and areas of heated argument, but everyone is telling a story of what they saw. Science is a collection of personal narratives.

A story of Sherrington's sums up Cajal's restless eye and passion and, I feel, defines his personality and greedy interest in the patterns of life. During his two-week stay in England in 1894, Cajal expressed how surprised he was that a city like London was so quiet. Where were the factories and industry that employed and fed its residents? At this point London was by far the largest city on the planet, but it seemed to Cajal, raised in small towns, that something was not quite right.

If you have ever been to London Bridge in the rush hour, you will see the driving mass of humanity that is London's lifeblood. Where I sit in my laboratory now is five minutes from the flood of people, packed together in phalanxes, who cross the bridge each day.

It was no different in 1894 and Charles Sherrington decided to show Cajal how the city worked by taking him to London Bridge during the surge of early-morning commuters.

Cajal was awestruck. The complexity, the self-organising streams of pedestrians, the urgency were compelling. I can imagine him standing there and watching, absorbing the details, gripped by the scene. The mass of human stories, each individual a universe of experience. He returned the next day and the next to watch, fascinated.

Perhaps, Santiago Ramón y Cajal saw more glimpses of the landscape on the other side of the fence, and was more passionate about the whole that he had pieced together in his mind. He had conviction, he knew he was right, he had imagined the landscape and it made sense. It turns out that he was right (or almost right) every time. He felt in his core the way that information flowed, how brain cells contacted each other, how and why they grew the way they grew, and the possibilities that his landscape gave for a mind that roams there.[i]

But what of the brain itself – what is its story?

To me there is a compelling and obvious truth at the heart of the story of brain cells. The landscape of the brain is an alien intelligence speaking a language we do not understand. It does, however, take the time to communicate to us in a simplified and rational way, translating a jumble of individual brain cell narratives such as the crowds on London Bridge into a simple scene. The brain talks to us in a way that patches up inconsistencies and holes in perceptions, losses of memory and incoherencies. For the most part it is telling us a story that makes sense. The story is reassuring, it calms our anxiety. Optical illusions are avoided, faces are recognised, changes in air pressure become words, fragments of co-activated activity become memories.

And even when the information is compromised, the brain does its best to keep us happy; we lose a chunk of our retina, the brain fills the gaps. We can't recognise a face; well then, hair colour and voice will do the job. The memories of facts become blurred and we make new memories that are just as compelling, just as genuine, even if others disagree. Perhaps it is only in disease or in our dreams that the brain as a storyteller begins to be less convincing. It pulls together associations, places, people, actions, and gives us a story that doesn't quite work. Despite the effort, the narrative thread is weaving dangerously, drunkenly at times. It's enough to know, if we are healthy, that this is a story not quite to be trusted.

The storytelling brain is the conscious brain and perhaps it is in the realm of the story that Sherrington's ghost, the psyche, finds its form. The mind is our story corner, where the pages are turned, and turned into urges and desires and fears. Stories allow us to order our predictions and expectations; what is going to be easy, difficult, rewarding, painful, joyous. The affordances of the world are a story told to us by the brain.

If we think this way for a moment, the quest to understand an alien brain or build an artificial intelligence is a search for alien and artificial stories. What is the narrative of the copepod central ganglion, experiencing the undersea world with its two photosensors scanning a horizontal view? What is the eight-dimensional story told by the octopus brain to the octopus self? Its tactile perspectives will be an unimaginable blur to our four-limbed brain, but what the octopus sees must be a coherent story of eight-limbed affordances.

And what then of artificial intelligence? The computer has undoubtedly surpassed our collective of brain cells in analytical power. Its architecture is designed to calculate, and the speed of its calculations grows faster and faster. The combinations of possibilities that can be weighed in any one femtosecond mean that a computer can begin to mimic the decisions of our own brain. It becomes difficult to tell the difference between a human and a computer in a blind trial. The human race is in peril.

Or is it? To my mind the most sophisticated and powerful computer, even the quantum computing of unlimited analytical speed, does not even approach the humble copepod until it can tell the story of its world. It has to want to fight, flee, feed or make love and choose between those decisions within its core. The poet, philosopher, psychiatrist and neuroscientist Warren McCulloch put these decisions, the heterarchy, at the heart of his artificial intelligence. The feeling of what it is to want or to be scared and the story of how to satisfy that want or mitigate that fear, and then making a choice on whether to act, are the decisions of the storytelling brain.

What makes the difference is the story. Cajal stands on London Bridge watching the swell of commuters in 1894 and returns day after day. Ten years earlier he looked down a microscope and saw, for the first time, the stunning and outlandish landscape of the brain cell. He looked at the scene and wanted to understand what was going on, why it was this way. What is the story here? *'Transfixed I could not turn my eye.'*

Notes

My first cell

i. Now Calle de Núñez de Arce.
ii. Now Calle de Augusto Figueroa.

Cell 1:
Purkinje's cell and the method of silhouettes

i. Notable scientists such as Gustaf Retzius were also in attendance, heightening Cajal's sense of discomfort.
ii. Deriving function from the structure of circuits is a compelling mix of engineering and architecture best described to my mind by these authors in particular: V. Braitenberg, *On the Texture of Brains* (Springer-Verlag, 1977); and P. Sterling and S. Laughlin, *Principles of Neural Design* (MIT Press, 2015).

Cell 3:
The astrocyte and neural glue

i. In Virchow's 1857 book *Cellular Pathology*. Virchow was host for many aspiring scientists including Charles Sherrington.

ii. Magendie was a ferocious vivisector, drawing criticism for his experiments on live animals from contemporary scientists and the general public. He possibly inspired H.G. Wells, who had studied zoology under T.H. Huxley and was a popular science writer, to create his science fiction novel *The Island of Doctor Moreau*.

Cell 4:
The sensory cell, Cajal's mistake and Freud's throwback

i. Adrian summed it up as follows. 'That particular day's work had all the elements that one could wish for . . . it didn't involve any particular hard work, or any particular intelligence on my part. It was one of those things which sometimes just happens in a laboratory if you stick apparatus together and see what results you get.'

ii. Nicolas André invented the term 'tic douloureux' in 1756 in the book *Observations pratiques sur les maladies de l'urethre, et sur plusiers faits convulsifs*.

iii. How the dendrite and the axon are stitched together in the cell body is a mystery. The story of this transformation has never grabbed much attention although, to me, it's quite remarkable in that it upsets the basic symmetry of a cell. There is some evidence that it is the product of both axon and dendrite becoming myelinated. (See Mudge, A.W., 'Schwann cells induce morphological transformation of sensory neurones in vitro', *Nature* 309 (1984), pp.367–9.) One theory to explain neuralgia is that the axons of sensory neurons are abandoned by the protective cells that normally wrap them in a healthy coating of fat, called myelin. The cells that wrap themselves around sections of the axons like rolled carpets are named after Theodor Schwann, one of the first scientists to propose that cells were the building blocks of both plants and animals. The sensory neuron is wrapped tightly with Schwann cells; these wrappings, rich in fatty myelin, provide an electrical insulation that speeds up the signals that run along its length.

iv. The fundamental paradox and problem that has repeatedly surfaced as a debate for scientists for more than a century is the position of the mesencephalic nucleus within the midbrain. All other sensory neurons find a position in a ganglion before they start making connections: their axons grow from the periphery to seek out other cells to share their information within the central nervous system.

v. Santiago Ramón y Cajal was also interested in reptiles and amphibians but delegated the study of these basal species to his now largely forgotten, but wildly adventurous, younger brother, Pedro Ramón y Cajal (1854–1950). Urged on by their tyrannical father, Pedro was destined to follow in the footsteps of his older brother to study medicine. However, he failed a single exam in his final year of school and rather than face the wrath of his father he fled to Bordeaux, stowing away on board a ship bound for South America at the age of seventeen, and disappeared. The next time anyone heard of his fate was when the Spanish consulate intervened to rescue Pedro from a death sentence handed out for stealing the horse and gun of a South American revolutionary leader (for whom Pedro had worked as a secretary). It emerged that Pedro had himself become a revolutionary, surviving a keelhauling, imprisonment, and wounds from armed skirmishes in Uruguay. He was rescued, repatriated and under duress returned to his medical studies. Pedro admitted that he studied the brain largely to confirm the findings of his more illustrious older brother. He was content to stay out of the limelight. However, the other scientists in the new field of comparative neuroscience were using the same species to unpick the evolutionary clues in brain cells that might explain evolution. With no fossil record of the spongy and delicate brains, the living descendants of ancestral creatures were and are the best hope of understanding the origins of brain and the organisation of its cells.

vi. In 1909, the thirty-eight-year-old neuroanatomist from Ohio, J.B. Johnston, laid down a challenge to future generations of anatomists: 'I have gone thus far with these speculations in order to show that very interesting problems lie here for other workers to determine more completely the morphology of these neurones in all classes of vertebrates, the disposition of their central processes, their origin and development and especially the history of the several processes, the axones and the motor collaterals. The size of the mesencephalic root and its constancy in all classes of vertebrates are sufficient proof of its importance and of the value of further studies along the lines indicated.'

vii. A young Sigmund Freud, enthralled with the new science of neuronal form, had also studied the unusual sensory cells embedded in the spinal cord in lampreys (the most primitive vertebrates) years before. He thought that these cells were neotenous – adult neurons that had maintained the characteristics of immature cells. Freud, S., 'Uber spinalganglien und ruckenmark des petromyzon', *Sitzungsberichte. Kaiserl. Akademie der Wissenschaften* (Wien), *Mathemat. Naturwiss. Classe* 75 (1878) pp.81–167.

Cell 5:
The leech neuron and the nerve net

i.   Two identical light twins exposed to different environments and recombined optically. If they have been treated the same, the superimposition is perfect, but any disruption appears as a ripple of interference.

ii. Wilhelm His was a great model maker and thinker about the shape changes in the embryo and formed a partnership with the Swiss firm of Ziegler to make accurate models, most famously of human embryos. The innovation that allowed this was a slicing machine called the microtome, invented by His, which allowed serial slices to be collected. The structures of the embryo were drawn and magnified using a camera lucida. The drawings were traced onto slabs of wax that were reassembled into giant embryos that could be held in two hands and passed between investigators. The Ziegler models still sit on dusty shelves in anatomy classrooms, modern students unaware of their age.

iii. This should be seen in the context of the emergence of a new science of sociology championed by Émile Durkheim in France.

iv. Nansen visited Golgi in Pavia in 1886 and published his account highlighting Golgi's contribution in 1887. Nansen was definitive in saying that there was a gap between nerve cells.

v.   This is the interpretation by a later writer, but Freud's explanation was that he wanted to deny a biographer (his later, imagined biographer) access to his manuscripts and thoughts (including cell biology) that he thought unworthy.

Cell 6:
A *universal brain cell*

i. I also collaborated with the artist Andrew Carnie. Together, we asked some of his non-science students to draw their impression of a neuron. What came out was a far more fluid and compelling set of pictures than the rigid and stereotyped pictures made by science students. They had the feeling of information flow and organic form but lacked the independent integrity of the single brain cell.

ii. Waldeyer presents an interesting tale of science anti-hero and was certainly a thorn in Cajal's side. He was an accomplished and eminent anatomist, but not so much an innovator as an appropriator and populariser. It seems that claiming the right to give the neuron its name reflected Waldeyer's sense of entitlement – an academic entitlement that was already becoming old-fashioned in the 1890s. He embodied discordant personal contrasts. He was affable and well liked, but he vehemently opposed women being admitted to medical school, and authored colonial-era anatomical publications that were facilitated by the appalling atrocities of African invasions by European powers, of which Waldeyer was not unaware. Waldeyer (von Waldeyer-Hartz after he received a peerage from the German Emperor) wanted his body to be preserved and examined. He believed that the difference between his right and left hands warranted some scientific exploration, but mostly it seemed to him that his brain might hold the clues to genius. This was not an unusual notion; as late as 1942, the renowned Egyptologist Sir William Flinders Petrie insisted that his head be preserved as a specimen for study. When Petrie died in Jerusalem, the Second World War delayed the return of his head to London but eventually it arrived at the Royal College of Surgeons where it remains today, although not on display.

iii. This detachment allowed Barker to drift rapidly away from the brain cell and towards a career that saw him lead the development of medical training and in particular scope research laboratories in medical schools. Shortly after the publication of *The Nervous System*, Barker travelled to Germany to work with Wilhelm His, but his interests had already moved back to medicine. Shortly before his prestigious invitation to head the anatomy department at the University of Chicago, he joined expeditions from Johns Hopkins to the Philippines and then to San Francisco (to investigate an apparent outbreak of bubonic plague). However, he was becoming increasingly interested in psychiatry and neurology and after three years in Chicago he returned to Baltimore, bringing with him the idea that research and teams of clinicians could accomplish far more than a single doctor on his own. Despite an enormous endowment from the Rockefeller Foundation with the explicit aim of bringing research-minded doctors like Barker into the medical school on a full-time basis, Barker, brought up in relative poverty, became in 1914, for the first time, a full-time clinician with a profitable practice.

Cell 7:
Betz's brain cell and the mapping of the cortex

i. What now for these precious specimens in a country that (at the time of writing) is again in the throes of conflict?

ii. The relative extent of cortical territory given over to, for example, a thumb (extensive) versus a little finger (much smaller) also matches how often we mistake which finger has been stroked when our eyes are closed (the thumb almost never), how prominently they are part of a phantom limb, and even to the frequency of their appearance in written English language (the little finger far less often). We name fingers but not toes, and the cortical representation is proportional to an importance that is functional and semantic. Halnan, C. and G.H. Wright, 'Fingers and toes in the body-image', *Acta Neurologica Scandinavica* 37 (1961) pp.50–61.

iii. Human layer V pyramidal cell dendrites can occasionally show pronounced asymmetries, extending into a neighbour's territory. As we grow older and more infirm, our Betz neurons begin to lose some of their structure. Their massive upwardly spiral-ling dendrite begins to topple and collapse. The horizontally stretching ropes of dendritic branches that wrap themselves around other cells falter and retract. It is a little like the cortex letting go bit by bit, relaxing into old age. Scheibel, M.E., U. Tomiyasu and A.B. Scheibel, 'The aging human Betz cell', *Experimental Neurology* 56 (1977) pp.598–609.

Cell 8:
The reticulothalamic cell and the seat of consciousness

i. The beautiful unusual, repeating patterns produced by X-ray crystallography spilled over into popular culture: the striking symmetry caught the imagination of both scientists and designers. The patterns produced by the crystal structure insulin, captured by Nobel laureate Dorothy Hodgkin (1910–1994), became the template for a wallpaper design at the Festival of Britain in 1951, joining a suite of fabrics inspired by atomic and microscopic images.

Cell 9:
The Scheibel cell and the heterarchy

i. In pictures, Warren Sturgis McCulloch appears with the long beard of a biblical prophet, clothed in the tweed of an Edwardian gentleman, with fierce, piercing eyes and an uncompromising stare. He was no ordinary neuroscientist – more a philosopher driven by a desire to achieve a comprehensive theory of mind, who tried to bridge the gap between the brain, engineering, mathematics and psychiatry and who is remembered chiefly as a pioneer of computer science.

ii. Pitts never completed a university degree but worked with eminent mathematicians and biophysicists. One of the more intriguing characters within neuroscience, he died in 1949 aged only forty-six, a compulsive reader and heavy drinker who had given up research some ten years earlier.

iii. McCulloch, however, cautioned, in verse, against any observer trying to deduce his reasoning or motives.

> When I am dead let no man say
> That had I lived, I had done so and so
> For I was always on an unknown way
> To mine own ends, the which they could not know.

Cell 10:
The motor neuron, a final common pathway and Sherrington's ghost

i. Sherrington shared his Nobel Prize with Edgar Adrian in 1932.

ii. Sherrington has at least five pictures of the reflex in his book *The Integrative Action of the Nervous System* (Cambridge University Press, 6th edn., 1947) pp.108, 150, 158, 202, 228.

iii. By this logic, Sherrington might well have argued that the adult sea squirt had 'lost its mind'. However, he strongly disagreed with the originator of dualistic conversations about mind and body, the French philosopher René Descartes (1596–1650), who privileged the psyche as a unique quality of humans while dogs and cattle were mere puppets of a series of reflex reactions to their environment.

iv. Sherrington's poetry was published late in his life (*The Assaying of Branbantius and Other Verse*, 1925).

Cell 10½:
The giant axon and the little yellow spot

i. Andrew was the half-brother of Aldous Huxley, although so much younger than the famous writer that he could not have been the inspiration for Theodor Gumbril, the inventor of the inflatable trousers in *Antic Hay* (Huxley's first novel, published in 1923) – a myth that my father had gleefully pedalled to me for many years.

ii. Sereni was a young man with an intense and restless energy. He had enrolled in university at sixteen, was a lieutenant commissioned in the First World War at seventeen, and a qualified doctor MD at twenty-four. He spent his twenty-fifth year in London at University College, working early mornings and late nights to gain as much time as he could in the laboratory, stretching his scholarship as far as he could. He returned, aged twenty-six, to head the physiology section at the Naples marine biology station. A committed anti-fascist, he died in mysterious circumstance, aged only thirty, in the fevered political atmosphere of Mussolini's Italy. JZ Young carried the squid giant axon back to England and then to North America where he became the most notable champion of cephalopod research. He also gave Hodgkin and Huxley the tool needed to unlock the action potential.

iii. I went to Oxford to meet up with Ray. He had been the Professor of Anatomy when I first started drawing brain cells and remained eminently approachable, always interested and a mine of information. It was a fiercely cold day and Ray suggested we meet near the University Parks for lunch in a canteen after he had finished teaching. By this point, he was living on his own quite modestly following an illustrious career that had taken him from London to Madison Wisconsin, Chicago and then to be the Dr Lee's Professor of Anatomy at Oxford, where I had first encountered him. Along the way he had tutored and mentored a succession of brilliant scientists.

I had come to commune, as many people have described their conversations with Ray. I wanted to ask him about the relationship between the cerebellum, thalamus and cortex, to test out my ideas (which he disagreed with) and draw on his depth of knowledge (which was vast). Looking back, I am not sure where I had got the idea from; it seems incredibly precocious in retrospect. I guess it was a feeling that somehow Ray had a parental indulgence, although I had never worked with him directly, that would accommodate poorly articulated questions and deep ignorance.

When I first met Ray, he encapsulated the stereotypical figure of the neuroanatomy professor of my subconscious student imagination. His office was high-ceilinged, spacious and had bookshelves filled with boxes upon boxes of slides. On his desk, instead of a computer, there was a microscope. Far from daunting, Ray always had a smile in the corner of his eye, as if everything I said was interesting, perhaps slightly amusing but always to be greeted with a benevolent, almost undetectable wink.

I had a peculiar sense that this had all happened before – an encounter repeated many times in the social structures of science as apprentice and savant conduct an awkward hand-off of knowledge: awkward in the allocation of roles that we may not want but that the situation dictates. My father was a medical student in the 1950s. He ran into his teacher, Hans Krebs, just after Krebs had received the Nobel Prize for Physiology for the discovery of the chemical pathway underlying energy production in the cell. My father was bright, but a little distracted by preparations for the new Edinburgh Festival and his penchant for partying. 'My dear David . . .' began Krebs, before walking down the South Parks Road. The soft-spoken laureate was describing to my dad how to focus and steer his scientific career. But in the noise of traffic, my father never heard a word. He thanked Hans Krebs as they separated, none the wiser. Fifty years later, here I was, retracing his exact steps with Ray.

I left what was to be our last meeting with the sense of being somewhat generously put in my place. My ideas were diametrically opposed to Ray's, and I have no reason to believe that he will not be proved correct in the fulness of time. I was, however, curious why Ray was still teaching dissection with cadavers to medical students in his late eighties on a cold weekday in a bleak Oxford. He explained that, apart from a good excuse to eat in the university staff club, he saw it as a duty and a privilege to pass on his learning for as long as he was able. He died later that year.

Epilogue

i. Was the bond between Cajal and his unlikely admirer, Charles Sherrington, something that grew from the search for this landscape? Cajal scanning the trees, drawing their branches and leaves, guessing at their root structure and growth; Sherrington, at arm's length, testing the landscape for its affordances but never losing himself in a forest of brain cells he could not have understood; both of them searching for and approaching an overall view, a complete picture.

References

1. Sherrington, C.S., 'Santiago Ramón y Cajal, 1852–1934', *Obituary Notices of Fellows of the Royal Society* 1(4) (1935).
2. Chorobski, J., 'Camillo Golgi 1843–1926', *Archives of Neurology & Psychiatry* 33 (1935) pp.163–70.
3. Clarke, E. and C.D. O'Malley, *The Human Brain and Spinal Cord: A Historical Study Illustrated by Writings from Antiquity to the Twentieth Century* (University of California Press, 1968) p.30.
4. Meek, J. and R. Nieuwenhuys, 'Palisade pattern of mormyrid Purkinje cells: a correlated light and electron microscopic study', *Journal of Comparative Neurology* 306 (1991) pp.156–92.
5. Stendell, W., 'Die Faseranatomie des Mormyridengehirns', *Abhandlungen der Senckenbergischen Naturforschenden Gesellschaft* 36 (1914).
6. Gregory, R.L., H.E. Ross and N. Moray, 'The curious eye of *Copilia*', *Nature* 201 (1964) p.1166–8.
7. Wolken, J.J. and R.G. Florida, 'The eye structure and optical system of the crustacean copepod, *Copilia*', *Journal of Cell Biology* 40 (1969) pp.279–85.

8. Rueda Esteban, R.J. et al., 'Corrosion casting, a known technique for the study and teaching of vascular and duct structure in anatomy', *International Journal of Morphology* 35 (2017) pp.1147–53.

9. Narat, J.K., J.A. Loef and M. Narat, 'On the preparation of multicolored corrosion specimens', *Anatomical Record* 64 (1936) pp.155–60.

10. Ndubaku, U. and M.E. de Bellard, 'Glial cells: old cells with new twists', *Acta Histochemica* 110 (2008) pp.182–95.

11. Navarrete, M. and A. Araque, 'The Cajal school and the physiological role of astrocytes: a way of thinking', *Frontiers in Neuroanatomy* 8 (2014) p.33.

12. Mestre, H. et al., 'Flow of cerebrospinal fluid is driven by arterial pulsations and is reduced in hypertension', *Nature Communications* 9 (2018) 4878.

13. Xie, L. et al., 'Sleep drives metabolite clearance from the adult brain', *Science* 342 (2013) pp.373–7.

14. Lucas, K., 'The "all or none" contraction of the amphibian skeletal muscle fibre', *Journal of Physiology* 38 (1909) p.113.

15. Hodgkin, A., 'Edgar Douglas Adrian, Baron Adrian of Cambridge, 30 November 1889 – 4 August 1977', *Biographical Memoirs of Fellows of the Royal Society* 25 (1979) pp.1–73.

16. Stookey, B. and J. Ransohoff, *Trigeminal Neuralgia: Its History and Treatment* (Thomas, 1959).

17. Pearce, J., 'Trigeminal neuralgia (Fothergill's disease) in the 17th and 18th centuries', *Journal of Neurology, Neurosurgery & Psychiatry* 74 (2003) p.1688.

18. Johnston, J.B., 'The radix mesencephalica trigemini',

Journal of Comparative Neurology and Psychology 19 (1909) pp.593–644.

19. Edwards, J.S. and R. Huntford, 'Fridtjof Nansen: from the neuron to the North Polar Sea', *Endeavour* 22 (1998) pp.76–80.

20. Barker, L.F., *The Nervous System and Its Constituent Neurones: Designed for the Use of Practitioners of Medicine and of Students of Medicine and Psychology* (D. Appleton, 1899).

21. Daston, L. and P. Galison, *Objectivity* (Zone Books, 2007).

22. Cajal, S. R. y, *Recollections of My Life* (MIT Press, 1989) p.104.

23. Capote, T., *Portraits and Observations: The Essays of Truman Capote* (Modern Library, 2013) p.270.

24. Cajal, S. R. y, *Precepts and Counsels on Scientific Investigation Stimulants of the Spirit* (Pacific Press, 1951) p.76.

25. Kushchayev, S.V. et al., 'The discovery of the pyramidal neurons: Vladimir Betz and a new era of neuroscience', *Brain* 135 (2012) pp.285–300.

26. Ibid.

27. Glickstein, M. and D. Whitteridge, 'Tatsuji Inouye and the mapping of the visual fields on the human cerebral cortex', *Trends in Neurosciences* 10 (1987) pp.350–3.

28. Kutia, S. et al., 'Famous morphologists who died young', *Journal of Health Sciences* 3 (2013) pp.347–58.

29. Guillery, R.W., 'Observations of synaptic structures: origins of the neuron doctrine and its current status', *Philosophical Transactions of the Royal Society B: Biological Sciences* 360 (2005) pp.1281–307.

30. Scheibel, M.E. and A.B. Scheibel, 'Structural substrates for integrative patterns in the brain stem reticular core',

in H.H. Jasper et al. (eds), *Reticular Formation of the Brain* (Little, Brown, 1958) pp.31–55.

31. Faraguna, U. et al., 'Editorial: The functional anatomy of the reticular formation', *Frontiers in Neuroanatomy* 13 (2019) p.55.

32. McCulloch, W.S. and W. Pitts, 'A logical calculus of the ideas immanent in nervous activity', *Bulletin of Mathematical Biophysics* 5 (1943) pp.115–33.

33. Kilmer, W.L., W.S. McCulloch and J. Blum, 'A model of the vertebrate central command system', *International Journal of Man–Machine Studies* 1 (1969) pp.279 –309.

34. Sherrington, C., *The Integrative Action of the Nervous System* (Cambridge University Press, 1947).

35. De Leo, A., 'Enrico Sereni: research on the nervous system of cephalopods', *Journal of the History of the Neurosciences* 17 (2008) pp.56–71.